T0264029

Sepsis

Editors

JENNIFER B. MARTIN
JENNIFER E. BADEAUX

CRITICAL CARE NURSING CLINICS OF NORTH AMERICA

www.ccnursing.theclinics.com

Consulting Editor
JAN FOSTER

September 2018 • Volume 30 • Number 3

ELSEVIER

1600 John F. Kennedy Boulevard • Suite 1800 • Philadelphia, Pennsylvania, 19103-2899

http://www.theclinics.com

CRITICAL CARE NURSING CLINICS OF NORTH AMERICA Volume 30, Number 3
September 2018 ISSN 0899-5885, ISBN-13: 978-0-323-64147-0

Editor: Kerry Holland
Developmental Editor: Laura Fisher

© 2018 Elsevier Inc. All rights reserved.

This periodical and the individual contributions contained in it are protected under copyright by Elsevier, and the following terms and conditions apply to their use:

Photocopying
Single photocopies of single articles may be made for personal use as allowed by national copyright laws. Permission of the Publisher and payment of a fee is required for all other photocopying, including multiple or systematic copying, copying for advertising or promotional purposes, resale, and all forms of document delivery. Special rates are available for educational institutions that wish to make photocopies for non-profit educational classroom use. For information on how to seek permission visit www.elsevier.com/permissions or call: (+44) 1865 843830 (UK)/(+1) 215 239 3804 (USA).

Derivative Works
Subscribers may reproduce tables of contents or prepare lists of articles including abstracts for internal circulation within their institutions. Permission of the Publisher is required for resale or distribution outside the institution. Permission of the Publisher is required for all other derivative works, including compilations and translations (please consult www.elsevier.com/permissions).

Electronic Storage or Usage
Permission of the Publisher is required to store or use electronically any material contained in this periodical, including any article or part of an article (please consult www.elsevier.com/permissions). Except as outlined above, no part of this publication may be reproduced, stored in a retrieval system or transmitted in any form or by any means, electronic, mechanical, photocopying, recording or otherwise, without prior written permission of the Publisher.

Notice
No responsibility is assumed by the Publisher for any injury and/or damage to persons or property as a matter of products liability, negligence or otherwise, or from any use or operation of any methods, products, instructions or ideas contained in the material herein. Because of rapid advances in the medical sciences, in particular, independent verification of diagnoses and drug dosages should be made.

Although all advertising material is expected to conform to ethical (medical) standards, inclusion in this publication does not constitute a guarantee or endorsement of the quality or value of such product or of the claims made of it by its manufacturer.

Critical Care Nursing Clinics of North America (ISSN 0899-5885) is published quarterly by Elsevier Inc., 360 Park Avenue South, New York, NY 10010-1710. Months of issue are March, June, September, and December. Business and Editorial Offices: 1600 John F. Kennedy Blvd., Suite 1800, Philadelphia, PA 19103-2899. Periodicals postage paid at New York, NY and additional mailing offices. Subscription prices are $155.00 per year for US individuals, $385.00 per year for US institutions, $100.00 per year for US students and residents, $200.00 per year for Canadian individuals, $483.00 per year for Canadian institutions, $230.00 per year for international individuals, $483.00 per year for international institutions and $115.00 per year for Canadian and international students/residents. To receive student/resident rate, orders must be accompanied by name of affiliated institution, data of term, and the *signature* of program/residency coordinator on institution letterhead. Orders will be billed at individual rate until proof of status is received. Foreign air speed delivery is included in all *Clinics* subscription prices. All prices are subject to change without notice. **POSTMASTER:** Send address changes to *Critical Care Nursing Clinics of North America*, Elsevier Health Sciences Division, Subscription Customer Service, 3251 Riverport Lane, Maryland Heights, MO 63043. **Customer Service: 1-800-654-2452 (US and Canada); 314-447-8871 (outside US and Canada). Fax:** 314-447-8029. **E-mail:** JournalsCustomerService-usa@elsevier.com **(for print support) and** JournalsOnlineSupport-usa@elsevier.com **(for online support).**

Reprints. For copies of 100 or more of articles in this publication, please contact the Commercial Reprints Department, Elsevier Inc., 360 Park Avenue South, New York, New York, 10010-1710; Tel.: 212-633-3874, Fax: 212-633-3820, and E-mail: reprints@elsevier.com.

Critical Care Nursing Clinics of North America is covered in *MEDLINE/PubMed (Index Medicus), International Nursing Index, Nursing Citation Index, Cumulative Index to Nursing and Allied Health Literature,* and *RNdex Top 100.*

Contributors

CONSULTING EDITOR

JAN FOSTER, PhD, APRN, CNS
Formerly, Associate Professor, College of Nursing, Texas Woman's University, Houston, Texas; Currently, President, Nursing Inquiry and Intervention, Inc, The Woodlands, Texas

EDITORS

JENNIFER B. MARTIN, DNP, CRNA, APRN
Instructor, Nurse Anesthesia Program, LSU Health New Orleans School of Nursing, New Orleans, Louisiana

JENNIFER E. BADEAUX, DNP, CRNA, APRN
Assistant Professor, Nurse Anesthesia Program, LSU Health New Orleans School of Nursing, New Orleans, Louisiana

AUTHORS

MARIE ADORNO, PhD, APRN, CNS, RNC
Assistant Professor of Clinical Nursing, LSU Health New Orleans School of Nursing, The Louisiana Center for Promotion of Optimal Health Outcomes: A Joanna Briggs Institute Centre of Excellence, New Orleans, Louisiana

JENNIFER E. BADEAUX, DNP, CRNA, APRN
Assistant Professor, Nurse Anesthesia Program, LSU Health New Orleans School of Nursing, New Orleans, Louisiana

KENDRA M. BARRIER, PhD, MSN, RN
Assistant Dean for Student Services, Instructor of Clinical Nursing Education, LSU Health New Orleans School of Nursing, New Orleans, Louisiana

LAURA S. BONANNO, DNP, CRNA, APRN
PhD Candidate, Director, Nurse Anesthesia Program, Associate Professor of Clinical Nursing, LSU Health Sciences Center School of Nursing, New Orleans, Louisiana

DENISE M. DANNA, DNS, RN, NEA-BC, CNE, FACHE
Chief Nursing Officer, University Medical Center New Orleans, New Orleans, Louisiana

ALISON H. DAVIS, PhD, RN, CHSE
Assistant Professor of Nursing, LSU Health Sciences Center School of Nursing, New Orleans, Louisiana

JUANITA L. DEROUEN, DNP, APRN, CRNA
Department of Anesthesia, Memorial Hospital at Gulfport, Gulfport, Mississippi

LEANNE H. FOWLER, DNP, MBA, AGACNP-BC, CCRN, CNE
Director of Nurse Practitioner Programs, Coordinator of Adult-Gerontology Acute Care
NP Concentration, LSU Health New Orleans School of Nursing, New Orleans, Louisiana

SHERRI P. HAYES, MSN, RN, CCRN
Instructor of Nursing, LSU Health Sciences Center School of Nursing, New Orleans,
Louisiana

JESSICA LANDRY, DNP, FNP-BC
Coordinator of Primary Care Family Nurse Practitioner Program, Nursing, LSU Health
New Orleans School of Nursing, New Orleans, Louisiana

JENNIFER MANNING, DNS, APRN, ACNS-BC, CNE
Associate Dean for Undergraduate Programs, LSU Health Sciences Center School of
Nursing, New Orleans, Louisiana

JENNIFER B. MARTIN, DNP, CRNA, APRN
Instructor, Nurse Anesthesia Program, LSU Health New Orleans School of Nursing,
New Orleans, Louisiana

SHANNON PERKINS, MSN, APRN, NNP-BC
Assistant Professor of Nursing, Delgado Community College-Charity School of Nursing,
New Orleans, Louisiana

MONICA SCHEEL, MSN, RN
Instructor of Nursing, Delgado Community College-Charity School of Nursing,
New Orleans, Louisiana

TODD TARTAVOULLE, DNS, APRN, CNS-BC
Program Director for the Baccalaureate Program, LSU Health New Orleans School of
Nursing, New Orleans, Louisiana

Contents

The Surviving Sepsis Campaign: International Guidelines for Management of Sepsis and Septic Shock: 2016 provides updated recommendations, rationales, and evidence tables for best care of patients with sepsis. "Sepsis is a life-threatening organ dysfunction caused by a dysregulated host response to infection. Septic shock (sepsis-3) is a subset of sepsis with circulatory and cellular/metabolic dysfunction associated with a higher risk of mortality than with sepsis alone." Sepsis and septic shock are major health care problems, affecting millions of people around the world each year. Early identification and management of sepsis and septic shock in the initial hours after sepsis develops improves outcomes.

Fluid resuscitation in the management of patients with sepsis and severe sepsis has been considered the standard of care for almost 2 decades. The rationale for fluid resuscitation is related to improvement in cardiac output and organ perfusion. Recent research evidence challenges the use of fluid resuscitation in patients diagnosed with sepsis. Research is needed to determine the timing of fluid administration, as well as the volume and type of fluid to achieve positive patient outcomes. This article discusses the pros and cons of early fluid administration in the management of patients with sepsis.

Medical care progress has enabled more patients in the intensive care unit to survive critical illnesses and return to daily living. This shift in survival rates has shed new light on the emotional consequences of this experience. For patients surviving an intensive care unit stay, posttraumatic stress disorder has been identified in approximately 9% to 27% compared with 7% of the general US population. Practitioners have an important role to play in early identification of patients experiencing signs and symptoms of this disorder. Timely interventions and treatment may reduce the incidence of physical and psychological comorbid conditions.

disturbing mortality rates, that accompany this condition. Sepsis is one of the costliest conditions billed to all payer groups: Medicare, Medicaid, private insurance, and uninsured patients. Health care organizations have implemented multiple strategies and best practices to improve the outcomes of patients with a diagnosis of sepsis.

CRITICAL CARE NURSING
CLINICS OF NORTH AMERICA

THE CLINICS ARE AVAILABLE ONLINE!
Access your subscription at:
www.theclinics.com

Preface

Sepsis: Special Considerations, Management, and Treatment for Diverse Patient Populations

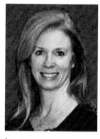 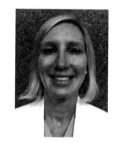

Jennifer B. Martin, DNP, CRNA   Jennifer E. Badeaux, DNP, CRNA
Editors

In the United States, sepsis and severe sepsis continue to be the leading causes of death and the most common cause of death among critically ill patients in noncoronary intensive care units (ICUs). The incidence of severe sepsis is estimated to be 300 cases per 100,000 people in the United States population, with approximately half of these cases occurring outside of an ICU setting. Recently reported data speculate an annual cost of $14 to 16 billion for hospital care of patients with septicemia.

Special considerations and management of care for a diverse patient population with sepsis should be current and evidence based. The ICU practitioner must remain well informed of standard care for patients with sepsis and consider alternatives and adjunct treatments by integrating innovative techniques. Interprofessional education and collaboration, with the use of high-fidelity simulation, can offer ICU practitioners improved knowledge and confidence in management of patients with sepsis. The ICU setting can be a traumatic experience, and therefore, collaboration among health care providers is essential for the well-being of patients with sepsis.

Jennifer B. Martin, DNP, CRNA
Nurse Anesthesia Program
Louisiana State University
Health New Orleans School of Nursing
1900 Gravier Street
New Orleans, LA 70112, USA

Crit Care Nurs Clin N Am 30 (2018) ix–x
https://doi.org/10.1016/j.cnc.2018.06.001
0899-5885/18/© 2018 Published by Elsevier Inc.

Jennifer E. Badeaux, DNP, CRNA
Nurse Anesthesia Program
Louisiana State University
Health New Orleans School of Nursing
1900 Gravier Street
New Orleans, LA 70112, USA

E-mail addresses:
jmar19@lsuhsc.edu (J.B. Martin)
jbadea@lsuhsc.edu (J.E. Badeaux)

Summary of the 2016 International Surviving Sepsis Campaign
A Clinician's Guide

Kendra M. Barrier, PhD, MSN, RN

KEYWORDS

- Sepsis • Septic shock • Surviving Sepsis Campaign (SSC) International Guidelines
- Organ dysfunction • Management • Clinician

KEY POINTS

- Facilitate earlier recognition.
- Sepsis and septic shock are medical emergencies; therefore, recommendations for treatment and resuscitation should start immediately.
- Timely intervention and management of patient with sepsis/septic shock improves outcomes; each hour delay in administration of appropriate antimicrobials is associated with a measurable increase in mortality.

INTERNATIONAL SEPSIS GUIDELINES 2016

The Surviving Sepsis Campaign (SSC): International Guidelines for Management of Sepsis and Septic Shock: 2016 provides updated recommendations, rationales, and evidence tables for best care of patients with sepsis.[1] "Sepsis is a life-threatening organ dysfunction caused by a dysregulated host response to infection.[2–4] Septic shock (sepsis-3) is a subset of sepsis with circulatory and cellular/metabolic dysfunction associated with a higher risk of mortality than with sepsis alone."[4] Patients with septic shock can be clinically identified by vasopressor requirement to maintain a mean arterial pressure (MAP) of 65 mm Hg or greater and a serum lactate level greater than 2 mmol/L (>18 mg/dL) in the absence of hypovolemia.[2] Vasopressor requirement and elevated lactate levels are associated with hospital mortality rates greater than 40%.[2] Patients with sepsis are 8 times more likely to die during hospitalization.[5] Sepsis and septic shock are major health care problems, affecting millions of people around the world each year and killing as many as 1 in 4 and often more.[6–8] Early identification and evidence-based management of sepsis and septic shock in the initial

Disclosure Statement: The author has nothing to disclose.
Nursing, Louisiana State University Health New Orleans, School of Nursing, 1900 Gravier Street, Suite 4C1, New Orleans, LA 70112, USA
E-mail address: kbarri@lsuhsc.edu

Crit Care Nurs Clin N Am 30 (2018) 311–321
https://doi.org/10.1016/j.cnc.2018.04.001
0899-5885/18/© 2018 Elsevier Inc. All rights reserved.
ccnursing.theclinics.com

hours after sepsis develops, improves outcomes as much as polytrauma, myocardial infarction, or stroke.[1]

The SSC is the leading organization responsible for educating health care professionals on the most current scientific evidence on the timely and appropriate treatment. The 2016 SSC guidelines were generated by 55 international experts, with expertise in specific aspects of sepsis, formulating the executive and steering committees, with 2 guideline committees, the oversight group and the group heads, and[1,2] lastly, the Grading of Recommendations Assessment, Development, and Evaluation (GRADE) methodology group. The panel consisted of 5 sections: hemodynamics, infection, adjunctive therapies, metabolic, and ventilation.[1] The GRADE system assessed the quality of evidence from high to very low, and formulated recommendations as weak or strong, or when a best practice statement (BPS) was warranted.[1,9] The BPS represent ungraded strong recommendations and are used under strict criteria, when the benefit or harm is equivocal; meaning the new guidelines are guided by dynamic variables and ongoing evaluation of clinical response to treatment.[1] The GRADE method was applied in selecting only outcomes that were considered critical from the patient's perspective, based on 6 categories: (1) risk of bias, (2) inconsistency, (3) indirectness, (4) imprecision, (5) publication bias, and (6) other criteria, followed by assessment of the balance between benefit and harm, patients' values and preferences, cost and resources, and feasibility and acceptability of the intervention.[9] The Surviving Sepsis Guideline panel provided 93 statements, 32 strong, 39 weak, 18 best practice statements, and 4 unanswered questions, on the early management and resuscitation of patients with sepsis or septic shock.[1] The guidelines are a resource document of 67 pages of recommendations, rationales, evidence tables, and 655 references with approaches to treat the sepsis patient from initial diagnosis, resuscitation, antimicrobial therapy, source control, fluid/vasoactive therapy, and progressing through organ support and adjunctive therapy recommendations.[8] The recommendations are guidelines and are not intended as standards of care, but more of an individualized, "patient-centered" approach guide.

The 2016 consensus eliminated the terms "severe sepsis" and "systemic inflammatory response syndrome" (SIRS). Components of SIRS include tachycardia, tachypnea, hyperthermia, and abnormalities in peripheral white blood cell count.[10,11-] Previous studies have shown the presence of SIRS is nearly ubiquitous in hospitalized patients and occurs in benign conditions, both related to and not related to infection, and not adequately specific to the diagnosis of sepsis.[10] The new definitions focus on organ dysfunction and hypoperfusion in the presence of infection, than on inflammation, specifically SIRS.[2] Furthermore, the term "severe sepsis" is also no longer recommended.[2] Singer and colleagues[2] (2016) stated severe sepsis is hard to define clinically and is not helpful in guiding clinical interventions. Clinically, the septic shock subset includes patients with refractory hypotension despite adequate fluid resuscitation requiring vasoactive medications to maintain an MAP greater than 65 mm Hg. With an understanding of sepsis and the pathobiology of this life-threatening condition, it is essential that the clinician stay abreast of the changes to sepsis management with the most updated guidelines. There were numerous important changes and major advances made in the revised guidelines; initial resuscitation and antibiotic therapy are the domains with the most important changes and advances.[12]

The patient with sepsis could have any or all of the following symptoms related to infection: altered mental status (AMS); tachycardia (heart rate [HR] >90 beats/min); hypotension (systolic blood pressure [SBP] <90 beats/min, MAP <90 mm Hg, or SBP decrease >40 mm Hg); cough; dyspnea (respiratory rate [RR] greater than

22 breaths/min); temperature (T) greater than 38.3°C or less than 36°C; and a decreased capillary refill, cyanosis, or mottling. How does the clinician provide patient-centered care to the sepsis/septic shock patient, decreasing mortality? A summary of the approaches to treat the sepsis patient from initial diagnosis, resuscitation, antimicrobial therapy, source control, fluid/vasoactive therapy, and progressing through organ support and adjunctive therapy recommendations and best practice statements with a focus on interventions most pertinent to the clinician is discussed later.[8]

Screening for Sepsis, Performance Improvement, and Diagnosis

Performance improvement plans for hospitals and hospital systems for sepsis, including screening for acutely ill, high-risk patients, are associated with improved patient outcomes.[1,13] New guidelines recommend clinicians assess patients in the intensive care unit (ICU) with a diagnosed or suspected infection.[14] Sepsis screening has also been associated with decreased mortality.[1] Clinical screenings of organ dysfunction of in-hospital patients can be represented by increase in the Sequential (sepsis-related) Organ Failure Assessment (SOFA) score (**Box 1**). The SOFA score grades abnormalities by organ system and accounts for clinical interventions. Specific laboratory variables such as Pao_2, platelet count, creatinine level, and bilirubin level are needed for computation.[2] A Glasgow Coma Scale (GCS), MAP, urine output (u/o), and administration of vasopressors (type/dose/rate) are also needed.[4] The selection of variables and cutoff values were developed by consensus.[2] A patient diagnosed or suspected infection with an increase of 2 points or more from the baseline SOFA score meets criteria for sepsis.[14] An increased SOFA score is associated with mortality rates greater than 10%.[2]

The quick SOFA (qSOFA) is used to rapidly assess patients in the emergency department (ED) or admitted to the medical/surgical unit, or primary care/urgent care with an infection, and to identify patients at risk for clinical decline and sepsis-related organ dysfunction[1,2] (**Box 2**). In the presence of any 2 qSOFA criteria, the clinician should start thinking sepsis and prompt further evaluation.

Once screened with SOFA or qSOFA, the presence of a suspected infection triggers the clinician to start the implementation of the SSC bundle. The bundle is a core set of recommendations that are the cornerstone of sepsis performance improvement programs, aimed at improving management, lower mortality rates, and shorter length of stays (LOS).[1]

Box 1
SOFA

Respirations (Pao_2/Fio_2 ratio)

Coagulation (platelet count)

Liver function (bilirubin level)

Cardiovascular system (MAP)

Central nervous system (GCS)

Renal system (creatinine level or u/o)

Abbreviations: GCS, Glasgow Coma Scale; Pao_2/Fio_2 ratio, partial pressure of oxygen and fraction of inspired oxygen; u/o, urine output.

Box 2
qSOFA

RR >22 breaths/min

AMS

SBP ≤100 mm Hg

Note: Nurses should know the patient's baseline and be aware of other variables that could potentially affect qSOFA score (dementia, baseline low systolic blood pressure).

- Remarks: obtain 2 sets of blood cultures, aerobic and anaerobic, before antibiotic administration; at least one set from a peripheral site and the other from vascular access device, if present.
  - There should not be any substantial delay starting the antimicrobials.

Initial Resuscitation

- BPS: recognize that sepsis and septic shock are medical emergencies
- Initial treatment and fluid resuscitation should start immediately for stabilization of sepsis-induced hypoperfusion
  - Sepsis-induced hypoperfusion may be manifested by acute organ dysfunction and/or ± decreased blood pressure and increased serum lactate
- Administer 30 mL/kg of intravenous (IV) crystalloid fluids, given within first 3 hours of confirmed or suspected sepsis or sepsis-related hypoperfusion
  - The initial fluid bolus is often referred to as a fluid challenge
  - Fixed volume enables clinicians to initiate resuscitation while obtaining more specific information about the patient and while awaiting more precise measurements of hemodynamic status
- Additional fluids guided by frequent assessment of hemodynamic status
  - Remarks: reassessment of physiologic values (HR, BP, arterial oxygen saturation [SaO_2], RR, T, u/o, and other noninvasive or invasive monitoring, if available)
- BPS: further hemodynamic assessment (cardiac function)—to determine type of shock if examination does not lead to clear diagnosis
- Evaluate fluid responsiveness by dynamic over static variable:
  - Passive leg raise
  - Pulse or stroke volume variations induced by mechanical ventilations
- The nurse plays a critical role in monitoring appropriate fluid resuscitation, maintaining MAP greater than 65 mm Hg as the patient is transferred from ED to floor or ICU
- Measure lactate level; if elevated (>2 mmol/L), guide resuscitation to normalize lactate; an elevated lactate level is a marker of tissue hypoperfusion

Antimicrobial Therapy

- Administering IV antimicrobials as soon as possible after recognition and within 1 hour for both sepsis and septic shock
  - Each hour delay in administration of appropriate antimicrobials is associated with a measurable increase in mortality
  - Other studies show an adverse effect on secondary end points, LOS, acute kidney injury, acute lung injury, and organ injury assessed by SOFA score with increased delays

- Broad spectrum therapy with one or more antimicrobials to cover all likely pathogens, gram-positive and gram-negative organisms (including bacterial and potentially fungal or viral coverage)
- BPS: narrow empirical antimicrobial therapy once pathogen identification and sensitivities are established and/or clinical improvement is noted
- BPS: the recommendations are against sustained systemic antimicrobial prophylaxis in patients with severe inflammatory states of noninfectious origin (eg, severe pancreatitis, burn injury)
- BPS: optimize dosing strategies based on accepted pharmacokinetic/pharmacodynamics principles and specific drug properties in patients with sepsis and septic shock
- Empirical combination therapy (using at least 2 antibiotics of different antimicrobial classes) aimed at the most likely bacterial pathogens for the initial management of septic shock
- Do not routinely use combination therapy for ongoing treatment of most other serious infections, including bacteremia and sepsis without shock
  - Remarks: this does not preclude the use of multidrug therapy to broaden antimicrobial activity
- Combination therapy for the routine treatment of neutropenic sepsis/bacteremia is not recommended
  - Remarks: This does not preclude the use of multidrug therapy to broaden antimicrobial activity
- BPS: if combination therapy is used for septic shock, deescalation with discontinuation of combination therapy within the first few days in response to clinical improvement and/or evidence of infection resolution. This applies to both targeted (for culture-positive infections) and empirical (for culture-negative infections) combination therapy
- Seven to ten days is adequate antimicrobial treatment for most serious infections associated with sepsis and septic shock
  - Current guidelines recommend 7-day course of therapy for nosocomial pneumonia, both hospital-acquired and ventilator-associated (VAP)
- Longer courses are appropriate in patients who have a slow clinical response, undrainable foci of infection, bacteremia with *Staphylococcus aureus*, some fungal and viral infections, or immunologic deficiencies, including neutropenia
- Shorter courses are appropriate in some patients, particularly those with rapid clinical resolution following effective source control of intra-abdominal or urinary sepsis and those with anatomically uncomplicated pyelonephritis
- BPS: daily assessment for deescalation of antimicrobial therapy in patients with sepsis and septic shock
  - Studies have shown that daily prompting on the question of antimicrobial deescalation is effective and may be associated with improved mortality
- Measurement of procalcitonin levels can be used to support shortening the duration of antimicrobial therapy in sepsis patients
  - Procalcitonin levels can be used to support the discontinuation of empirical antibiotics in patients who initially seemed to have sepsis, but subsequently have limited clinical evidence of infection

Source Control

- BPS: specific anatomic diagnosis of infection requiring emergent source control should be identified or excluded as rapidly as possible in patients with sepsis or septic shock

- BPS: any required source control interventions should be implemented as soon as medically and logistically practical after diagnosis is made
- Prompt removal of IV access devices that are possible source of sepsis or septic shock after other vascular access has been established

Fluid Therapy

- BPS: a fluid challenge technique be applied where fluid administration is continued as long as hemodynamic factors continue to improve
- Administer crystalloids as the fluid of choice for initial resuscitation and subsequent intravascular volume replacement in patients with sepsis and septic shock
- Use either balanced crystalloids or saline for fluid resuscitation
- Use albumin in addition to crystalloids for initial resuscitation and subsequent intravascular volume replacement in patients with sepsis and septic shock, when patients require substantial amounts of crystalloids
- Using hydroxyethyl starches for intravascular volume replacement in patients with sepsis or septic shock is strongly not recommended
- Using crystalloids over gelatins when resuscitating patients with sepsis or septic shock

Vasoactive Medications

- Administer vasoactive medications if the patient remains hypotensive or if lactate remains elevated following the initial fluid challenge
- Norepinephrine as the first-choice vasopressor
  - Typically started at 2 to 5 mcg/min and titrated to MAP greater than 65 mm Hg
- Add either vasopressin (up to 0.03 U/min) or epinephrine to norepinephrine with the intent of raising MAP to target, or add vasopressin (up to 0.03 U/min) to decrease norepinephrine dosage
- Use dopamine as an alternative vasopressor agent to norepinephrine only in highly selected patients (eg, patients with low risk of tachyarrhythmias and absolute or relative bradycardia)
  - Using low-dose dopamine for renal protection is not recommend
- Use dobutamine in patients who show evidence of persistent hypoperfusion despite adequate fluid loading and the use of vasopressor agents
  - Remarks: if initiated, dosing should be titrated to an end point reflecting perfusion, and the agent reduced or discontinued in the face of worsening hypotension or arrhythmias
- An arterial catheter placed as soon as practical for all patients requiring vasopressors if resources are available

Corticosteroids

- IV hydrocortisone should not be used to treat septic shock patients if adequate fluid resuscitation and vasopressor therapy are able to restore hemodynamic stability
  - IV hydrocortisone at a dose of 200 mg/d, if hemodynamic stability is not achieved

Blood Products

- Red blood cell (RBC) transfusion occur only when hemoglobin concentration decreases to less than 7.0 g/dL in adults in the absence of extenuating circumstances, such as myocardial ischemia, severe hypoxemia, or acute hemorrhage
- Erythropoietin for treatment of anemia associated with sepsis is not recommended

- Fresh frozen plasma to correct clotting abnormalities in the absence of bleeding or planned invasive procedures are not recommended
- Prophylactic platelet transfusion when counts are less than 10,000/mm^3 (10 × 10^9/L) in the absence of apparent bleeding and when counts are less than 20,000/mm^3 (20 × 10^9/L) if the patient has a significant risk of bleeding
  - Higher platelet counts (≥50,000/mm^3 [50 × 10^9/L]) are advised for active bleeding, surgery, or invasive procedures

Immunoglobulins

- IV immunoglobulins in patients with sepsis or septic shock is not recommended

Blood Purification

- Use of blood purification techniques—no recommendation made

Anticoagulants

- Use of antithrombin for the treatment of sepsis and septic shock is not recommended
- Use of thrombomodulin or heparin for the treatment of sepsis or septic shock—no recommendation made

Mechanical Ventilation

- Target tidal volume of 6 mL/kg predicted body weight compared with 12 mL/kg in adult patients with sepsis-induced acute respiratory distress syndrome (ARDS)
- Use an upper limit goal for plateau pressures of 30 cm H$_2$O over higher plateau pressures in adult patients with sepsis-induced severe ARDS
- Use higher positive end-expiratory pressure (PEEP) over lower PEEP in adult patients with sepsis-induced moderate to severe ARDS
- Use recruitment maneuvers in adult patients with sepsis-induced, severe ARDS
- Use prone over supine position in adult patients with sepsis-induced ARDS and a Pao$_2$/Fio$_2$ ratio less than 150
- Using high-frequency oscillatory ventilation in adult patients with sepsis-induced ARDS is not recommended
- Use of noninvasive ventilation for patients with sepsis-induced ARDS—no recommendation made
- Use of neuromuscular blocking agents for less than or equal to 48 hours in adult patients with sepsis-induced ARDS and a Pao$_2$/Fio$_2$ ratio less than 150 mm Hg
- A conservative fluid strategy for patients with established sepsis-induced ARDS who do not have evidence of tissue hypoperfusion
- Use of beta-2 agonists for the treatment of patients with sepsis-induced ARDS without bronchospasm is not recommended
- Routine use of the pulmonary artery catheter for patients with sepsis-induced ARDS is not recommended
- Use lower tidal volumes over higher tidal volumes in adult patients with sepsis-induced respiratory failure without ARDS
- Mechanically ventilated sepsis patients be maintained with the head of the bed elevated between 30° and 45° to limit aspiration risk and to prevent the development of VAP
- Use spontaneous breathing trials in mechanically ventilated patients with sepsis who are ready for weaning
- Use a weaning protocol in mechanically ventilated patients with sepsis-induced respiratory failure who can tolerate weaning

Sedation and Analgesia

- BPS: continuous or intermittent sedation be minimized in mechanically ventilated sepsis patients, targeting specific titration end points

Glucose Control

- A protocolized approach to blood glucose management in ICU patients with sepsis, commencing insulin dosing when 2 consecutive blood glucose levels are greater than 180 mg/dL
  - This approach should target an upper blood glucose level less than or equal to 180 mg/dL than an upper target blood glucose level less than or equal to 110 mg/dL
- BPS: blood glucose values be monitored every 1 to 2 hours until glucose values and insulin infusion rates are stable, then every 4 hours thereafter in patients receiving insulin infusions
- BPS: glucose levels obtained with point-of-care testing of capillary blood be interpreted with caution because such measurements may not accurately estimate arterial blood or plasma glucose values
- Use of arterial blood than capillary blood for point-of-care testing using glucose meters if patients have arterial catheters

Renal Replacement Therapy

- Either continuous or intermittent renal replacement therapy (RRT) be used in patients with sepsis and acute kidney injury
- Use continuous therapies to facilitate management of fluid balance in hemodynamically unstable septic patients
- The use of RRT in patients with sepsis and acute kidney injury for increase in creatinine or oliguria without other definitive indications for dialysis is not recommended

Bicarbonate Therapy

- Use of sodium bicarbonate therapy to improve hemodynamics or to reduce vasopressor requirements in patients with hypoperfusion-induced lactic acidemia with pH greater than or equal to 7.15 is not recommended

Venous Thromboembolism Prophylaxis

- Pharmacologic prophylaxis (unfractionated heparin [UFH] or low-molecular-weight heparin [LMWH]) against venous thromboembolism (VTE) in the absence of contraindications to the use of these agents
- LMWH rather than UFH for VTE prophylaxis in the absence of contraindications to the use of LMWH
- Combination of pharmacologic VTE prophylaxis and mechanical prophylaxis, whenever possible
- Mechanical VTE prophylaxis when pharmacologic VTE is contraindicated

Stress Ulcer Prophylaxis

- Stress ulcer prophylaxis be given to patients with sepsis or septic shock who have risk factors for gastrointestinal (GI) bleeding
- Use either proton pump inhibitors or histamine-2 receptor antagonists when stress ulcer prophylaxis is indicated
- BPS: stress ulcer prophylaxis in patients without risk factors for GI bleeding is not recommended

Nutrition

- Administration of early parenteral nutrition alone or parenteral nutrition in combination with enteral feedings (but rather initiate early enteral nutrition) in critically ill patients with sepsis or septic shock who can be fed enterally is not recommended
- Administration of parenteral nutrition alone or in combination with enteral feeds (but to initiate IV glucose and advance enteral feeds as tolerated) over the first 7 days in critically ill patients with sepsis or septic shock for whom early enteral feeding is not feasible is not recommended
- Early initiation of enteral feeding than a complete fast or only IV glucose in critically ill patients with sepsis or septic shock who can be fed enterally
- Either early trophic/hypocaloric or early full enteral feeding in critically ill patients with sepsis or septic shock; if trophic/hypocaloric feeding is the initial strategy, then feeds should be advanced according to patient tolerance
- Use of omega-3 fatty acids as an immune supplement in critically ill patients with sepsis or septic shock is not recommended
- Routinely monitoring gastric residual volumes in critically ill patients with sepsis or septic shock is not recommended. However, measurement of gastric residuals in patients with feeding intolerance or who are considered to be at high risk of aspiration is recommended
  - Remarks: This recommendation refers to nonsurgical critically ill patients with sepsis or septic shock
- Use of prokinetic agents in critically ill patients with sepsis or septic shock and feeding intolerance
- Placement of postpyloric feeding tubes in critically ill patients with sepsis or septic shock with feeding intolerance or who are considered to be at high risk of aspiration
- Use of IV selenium, arginine, and glutamine to treat sepsis and septic shock is not recommended
- Use of carnitine for sepsis and septic shock had no recommendation made

Setting Goals of Care

- BPS: discuss goals of care and prognosis with patients and families
- Goals of care incorporated into treatment and end-of-life care planning, using palliative care principles where appropriate
- Address goals of care as early as feasible, but no later than within 72 hours of ICU admission

Because the guidelines could seem daunting, the author offers suggestions for a clearer understanding: review the comparison of recommendation tables of the 2012 and 2016 guidelines; review the new recommendations; read the rationales for the recommendations; and review the evidence tables and the grading of the evidence when the recommendation is contrary to expected.

The core of the sepsis improvement efforts are provided in the updated SSC bundle in response to new evidence. Using "bundles" simplifies the complex processes of the care of patients with severe sepsis by selecting a set of elements of care and when implemented as a group, have an effect on outcomes beyond implementing the individual elements alone.[15] The SSC Executive Committee has revised the improvement bundles as shown in **Boxes 3** and **4**.

The key strengths of the Surviving Sepsis Campaign (SSC): International Guidelines for Management of Sepsis and Septic Shock: 2016 provides new definitions for sepsis

---

Box 3
Surviving sepsis campaign bundle

To be completed within 3 hours:

1. Measure lactate level

2. Obtain blood cultures before administration of antibiotics

3. Administer broad spectrum antibiotics

4. Administer 30 mL/kg crystalloid for hypotension or lactate level greater than or equal to 4 mmol/L

To be completed within 6 hours:

5. Apply vasopressors (for hypotension that does not respond to initial fluid resuscitation) to maintain a mean arterial pressure (MAP) greater than or equal to 65 mm Hg

6. In the event of persistent hypotension after initial fluid administration (MAP <65 mm Hg) or if initial lactate level was greater than or equal to 4 mmol/L, reassess volume status and tissue perfusion and document findings according to **Box 4**

7. Remeasure lactate if initial lactate level is elevated

"Time of presentation" is defined as the time of triage in the ED or, if presenting from another care venue, from the earliest chart annotation consistent with all elements of severe sepsis or septic shock ascertained through chart review.

From Society of Critical Care Medicine. Surviving sepsis campaign: updated bundles in response to new evidence. Available at: http://www.survivingsepsis.org/SiteCollectionDocuments/SSC_Bundle.pdf; Reproduced from survivingsepsis.org. Copyright © 2018 the Society of Critical Care Medicine and the European Society of Intensive Care Medicine.

---

and septic shock and eliminated SIRS and severe sepsis. The updated recommendations, rationales, BPS, and comparison tables provide evidence for patient-centered care of adult patients with sepsis and septic shock. Nurses and interdisciplinary teams are able to improve patient outcomes by participating in hospital-wide performance improvement programs to implement/revise protocols using the new clinical criteria for septic shock that includes sepsis with fluid-unresponsive hypotension, serum

---

Box 4
Surviving sepsis campaign bundle continuation

Document reassessment of volume status and tissue perfusion with

Either
• Repeat focused examination (after initial fluid resuscitation) including vital signs, cardiopulmonary, capillary refill, pulse, and skin findings.

Or 2 of the following:
• Measure CVP
• Measure ScvO$_2$
• Bedside cardiovascular ultrasound
• Dynamic assessment of fluid responsiveness with passive leg raise or fluid challenge

Of note, the 6-hour bundle has been updated; the 3-hour SSC bundle is not affected.

Abbreviations: CVP, central venous pressure; ScvO$_2$, central venous oxygen saturation.
From Society of Critical Care Medicine. Surviving sepsis campaign: updated bundles in response to new evidence. Available at: http://www.survivingsepsis.org/SiteCollectionDocuments/SSC_Bundle.pdf; Reproduced from survivingsepsis.org. Copyright © 2018 the Society of Critical Care Medicine and the European Society of Intensive Care Medicine.

lactate level greater than 2 mmol/L, and the need for vasopressors to maintain MAP greater than 65 mm Hg or greater.[10,15] "The updated definitions and clinical criteria should replace previous definitions, offer greater consistency for epidemiologic studies and clinical trials, and facilitate earlier recognition and more timely management of patients with sepsis or at risk of developing sepsis."[2] Although the guidelines may be many things to different user groups, the SSC guidelines provide the core scientific evidence for sepsis management, in the ED, medical/surgical floor, or the ICU, with the intent of improving patient outcomes for the patient with a suspected infection, sepsis, or septic shock.

REFERENCES

1. Rhodes A, Evans LE, Alhazzani W, et al. Surviving sepsis campaign: international guidelines for the management of sepsis and septic shock: 2016. CritCare Med 2017;45:486–552.
2. Singer M, Deutschman CS, Seymour CW, et al. The third international consensus definitions for sepsis and septic shock (sepsis-3). JAMA 2016;315:801–10.
3. Shankar-Hari M, Phillips GS, Levy ML, et al, Sepsis Definitions Task Force. Developing a new definition and assessing new clinical criteria for septic shock: for the third international consensus definitions for sepsis and septic shock (sepsis-3). JAMA 2016;315:775–87.
4. Seymour CW, Liu VX, Iwashyna TJ, et al. Assessment of clinical criteria for sepsis: for the third international consensus definitions for sepsis and septic shock (sepsis-3). JAMA 2016;315:762–74.
5. Hall MJ, Williams SN, DeFrances CJ, et al. Inpatient care for septicemia or sepsis: a challenge for patients and hospitals. NCHS Data Brief No. 62. Centers for Disease Control and Prevention (CDC); 2011. Available at: https://www.cdc.gov/nchs/data/databriefs/db62.htm. Accessed December 22, 2017.
6. Angus DC, Linde-Zwirble WT, Lidicker J, et al. Epidemiology of severe sepsis in the United States: analysis of incidence, outcome, and associated costs of care. CritCare Med 2001;29:1303–10.
7. Dellinger RP. Cardiovascular management of septic shock. CritCare Med 2003; 31:946–55.
8. Martin GS, Mannino DM, Eaton S, et al. The epidemiology of sepsis in the United States from 1979 through 2000. N Engl J Med 2003;348:1546–54.
9. Guyatt GH, Oxman AD, Kunz R, et al. GRADE guidelines: 2. Framing the question and deciding on important outcomes. J ClinEpidemiol 2011;64:395–400.
10. Abraham E. New definitions for sepsis and septic shock continuing evolution but with much still to be done. JAMA 2016;315(8):757–9.
11. Dellinger RP, Schorr CA, Levy MM. A users' guide to the 2016 surviving sepsis guidelines. CritCare Med 2017;45(3):381–5.
12. De Backer D, Dorman T. Survivingsepsis guidelines a continuous move toward better care of patients with sepsis. JAMA 2017;317(8):807–8.
13. Dellinger PR. Forward.The future of sepsis performance improvement. CritCare Med 2015;43:1787–9.
14. Jacob JA. New sepsis diagnostic guidelines shift focus to organ dysfunction. JAMA 2016;315:739–40.
15. Critical Care Medicine. Available at: http://www.survivingsepsis.org/SiteCollection Documents/SSC_Bundle.pdf. Accessed December 22, 2017.

Early Administration of Intravenous Fluids in Sepsis
Pros and Cons

Laura S. Bonanno, DNP, CRNA, APRN*

KEYWORDS

- Sepsis • Septic shock • Intravenous fluid administration • Fluid resuscitation
- Early goal-directed resuscitation • Fluid management

KEY POINTS

- Sepsis is one of the leading causes of morbidity.
- Early administration of intravenous fluid is commonly used to decrease signs and symptoms of sepsis.
- The timing, volume, and type of fluid administered to patients diagnosed with sepsis impacts patient outcomes.
- Recent studies have challenged the notion that aggressive fluid resuscitation is beneficial in the management of sepsis.

INTRODUCTION

Sepsis is a potentially life-threatening response of the immune system to a severe infection.[1–4] It is a dynamic process requiring constant reassessment by nurses and other health care professionals.[5] Multiple definitions and terminologies are currently used for sepsis and septic shock, and this can lead to discrepancies in accurate reporting.[6] A taskforce that included experts in sepsis pathobiology, clinical trials, and epidemiology was convened by the Society of Critical Care Medicine and the European Society of Intensive Care Medicine to evaluate and update the current definitions for sepsis and septic shock. The revised definitions by Singer and colleagues[6] are commonly referred to as Sepsis-3:

Sepsis: "a life-threatening organ dysfunction caused by a dysregulated host response to infection."[6(p804)]

Organ dysfunction "represented by an increase in the Sequential Organ Failure Assessment (SOFA) score of 2 points or higher that is associated with a mortality

Disclosure: No conflict of interest.
Nurse Anesthesia Program, LSUHSC School of Nursing, 1900 Gravier Street, New Orleans, LA 70112, USA
* 217 Morningside Drive, Mandeville, LA 70448.
E-mail address: Lbonan@lsuhsc.edu

Crit Care Nurs Clin N Am 30 (2018) 323–332
https://doi.org/10.1016/j.cnc.2018.05.011
0899-5885/18/© 2018 Elsevier Inc. All rights reserved.

ccnursing.theclinics.com

greater than 10%."[6(p805)] The baseline SOFA score is assumed to be zero absent of any preexisting organ dysfunction. The quick SOFA (q SOFA) provides simple bedside criteria to identify adult patients and these criteria include[6(p805)]:

- Respiratory rate ≥22
- Altered mentation
- Systolic blood pressure ≤100 mm Hg

Septic Shock "a subset of sepsis in which particularly profound circulatory, cellular, and metabolic abnormalities are associated with a greater risk of mortality than with sepsis alone."[6(p805)] Associated with mortality rate greater than 40%.

- Vasopressor requirement to maintain mean arterial pressure (MAP) of 65 mm Hg or greater
- Serum lactate level >2 mmol/L (>18 mg/dL) in the absence of hypovolemia

The physiologic response, signs, and symptoms of sepsis can vary depending on the source and severity of the infection.[3] Common signs and symptoms include low blood pressure, fever, tachycardia, and tachypnea. Prompt detection and diagnosis of sepsis is critical because of the necessity to begin interventions early, which includes the administration of intravenous (IV) fluids, antibiotics, and vasoactive agents followed by source control.[4,7] A delay in beginning therapy correlates with an increased incidence of organ failure and higher mortality rate.[6]

The early management of sepsis is focused on the administration of antibiotics, IV fluids, and vasoactive agents, followed by controlling the source of the sepsis.[7] However, how to approach to the resuscitation of patients with septic shock is controversial. Although fluid resuscitation may be a necessity to manage life-threatening conditions in the early stages of shock, continuing resuscitation beyond that period may have detrimental effects.

In 2001, Rivers and colleagues[8] conducted a single-center randomized control trial (RCT) on the use of early goal-directed therapy (EGDT) to achieve certain hemodynamic optimization for the management of patients in the emergency room with septic shock. In this study, an EGDT 6-hour protocol for resuscitation was guided by specific hemodynamic goals targeting arterial pressure (MAP), central venous pressure (CVP), and central venous oxygen saturation (SVO2) of 70% or greater.[9] It is unclear whether the mortality benefits observed in the study by Rivers and colleagues[8] were the result of invasive hemodynamic monitoring and rigid protocol usage, or perhaps in early recognition and intervention afforded by the protocol.[4]

Since this 2001 study, there have been subsequent single and multicenter RCTs that suggest fluid administration is beneficial in septic shock. However, most of these studies show the benefits of a multimodal approach to the initial management of sepsis of which EGDT was central.[10] Fluid resuscitation is necessary at the early stages of septic shock to maintain hemodynamic stability. However, whether fluid resuscitation should continue beyond that period is questionable.[11] More recent studies suggest that aggressive fluid resuscitation results in volume overload and organ dysfunction, which has been associated with increased patient mortality.[7,10,11] Recently, 3 large, multicenter RCTs conducted in the United States, Australia, and the United Kingdom failed to find that EGDT decreased mortality.[9] In these RCTs designed to compare EGDT to usual care, the use of CVP did not improve mortality, and administration of IV fluids titrated to a selected CVP level has been implicated in volume overload.[9]

"Empiric fluid loading is the administration of a predetermined volume of fluid with the intent to ensure adequate organ perfusion."[12(p68)] In the study by Rivers and colleagues,[8] refractory hypotension was defined as systolic blood pressure lower than 90 mm Hg after a 20 to 30 mL/kg bolus. Based on the study by Rivers and colleagues,[8] the Surviving Sepsis Campaign (SSC) guidelines recommend an initial 30 mL/kg bolus of crystalloids for patients with sepsis and septic shock. In the 3 most recent RCTs that were conducted to study EGDT, patients received an average of 30 to 35 mL/kg fluid bolus before enrollment. The best practice appears to be individualized fluid therapy and administration of the fluid volume needed to treat hypovolemia.[10,12]

BACKGROUND
Incidence and Prevalence

Sepsis and septic shock affect millions of people globally with a mortality rate as high as 1 in 4.[3,4] Sepsis is one of the most common reasons that patients are admitted to intensive care units (ICU) and one of the most expensive conditions to treat in US hospitals.[2,7] Septic shock is also the most common form of shock found in patients admitted to ICUs.[13] The increased incidence is believed to be due to the aging population and complex comorbidities.[2,7] In the United States, sepsis affects more than 750,000 persons annually, and the prevalence of sepsis is 3 cases per 1000 persons.[1] Byrne and Van Haren[10] report that the mortality rate for patients with septic shock (most severe form of sepsis) is as high as 50%.

Risk Factors: age (elderly), severely malnourished, immunosuppressed.

Pathophysiology

In patients with septic shock, the major physiologic changes include "vasoplegic shock (distributive shock), myocardial depression, altered microvascular flow, and a diffuse endothelial injury." [7(p1407)] The pathophysiologic changes associated with shock play a central role in its management.[12] MAP is determined by cardiac output (CO) and systemic vascular resistance (SVR). "The primary determinants of CO are heart rate (HR) and stroke volume (SV)."[12(p60)] To maintain CO, blood is ejected from the left ventricle, traverses the circulatory system, returns to the right atrium and right ventricle, and then enters pulmonary circulation.[12] The Frank Starling curve is used to "illustrate the volume present in the left ventricle (LV) at the end of diastole (preload) and directly influences SV. Any increases in preload will result in an increase in SV until optimal preload is achieved and a plateau is reached."[12,14] Beyond that plateau point, additional preload, such as that administered as IV fluid will not be able to significantly increase SV leading to fluid overload resulting in impaired cardiac function, pulmonary edema, and interstitial edema.[12]

Lactate is produced as a result of adrenergic and inflammatory responses seen in sepsis.[11] Lactate during sepsis is not a marker of tissue hypoxia. Decreasing lactate marks the downregulation of the host inflammatory response, whereas improving capillary refill time and increasing urine output indicates improving organ perfusion.[11]

Assessing circulating blood volume

The heart and systemic vasculature is a complex system that preserves circulating volume effectiveness by mobilizing fluids via vasoconstriction, vasodilation, or increasing CO.[11] This physiologic response is dynamic and adapts continuously at a rapid rate; therefore, measuring CVP at one point in the day (static measure) provides an inaccurate assessment of overall fluid status.[11] CVP and pulmonary arterial occlusion pressure actually do not correlate with circulating blood volume.[11]

In septic shock, capillary leak and pathologic vasoplegia cause fluid depletion. However, continuing fluid administration will drive intravascular fluid into the interstitial space, producing marked tissue edema and disrupting vital oxygenation.[11] Therefore, early, adequate fluid resuscitation and vasopressors should be used in the treatment of patients with sepsis and a conservative fluid regimen should follow.[11]

Assessing fluid responsiveness

Fluid responsiveness is defined as "the state of preload reserve in which an increase in venous return results in an increase in cardiac output which corresponds to the ascending portion of the Frank Starling curve."[12(p68)] If SV or CO increases by approximately 15% in response to an increase in preload, this suggests the patient is responsive to fluids and will tolerate additional fluid administration.[12] If SV or CO changes <10% to 15%, this suggests additional fluids will not be beneficial to the patient, and the use of vasopressors should be considered.[12] It is important to note that only 50% of critically ill patients are responsive to fluid administration. Further, in patients who are fluid responders (respond to fluid boluses with an increase in CO), vasodilation with a fall in SVR has been observed and blood pressure may remain unchanged.[7] Although traditional physical examination findings to assess fluid responsiveness have been shown as poor indicators of fluid responsiveness, new methods and devices including invasive and noninvasive techniques provide measurements that are described as static (intermittent) or dynamic (continuous).[10]

Traditional static measurements, CVP, and pulmonary artery occlusive pressure do not accurately measure fluid responsiveness; therefore, these should not be used, especially in critically ill patients.[10] Further, 3 recent RCTs found no difference in patient outcomes with the use of CVP to guide fluid administration.[9] Dynamic measures have been consistently shown as superior to static measurements, which include fluid challenge, mini fluid challenge, and passive leg raise. The fluid challenge consists of infusion of 250 to 500 mL crystalloids over 10 minutes and if performed can prevent the harm of excessive fluid administration.[10] The passive leg-raising maneuver coupled with minimally invasive CO monitoring is useful in assessing volume responsiveness.[7,10] In patients who are not fluid responders, methods to minimize additional fluid administration should be considered, including discontinuation of maintenance fluids, minimizing carrier fluids, and removal of excess fluid via diuretics or ultrafiltration.[12]

Further, increased cardiac filling pressures consequent to large-volume resuscitation can cause extravascular lung water (EVLW), endothelial injury, capillary leak, and increased hydrostatic pressures resulting in less than 5% of infused crystalloids remaining intravascular within 3 hours after infusion.[7]

Fluid resuscitation in sepsis

In patients with any form of shock, fluid therapy is needed to improve microvascular blood flow and CO.[13] Fluid resuscitation continues to be the recommended first-line resuscitative therapy for patients with severe sepsis and septic shock.[10,12] This therapy is based on long history and familiarity with its use in resuscitation of other forms of shock; however, this might be based on an incorrect understanding of the pathophysiology of sepsis.[12] Early fluid resuscitation is necessary to maintain hemodynamic stability during the early stage of shock and resuscitation, but subsequent fluid administration should be guided by dynamic measurements of fluid responsiveness.[11,12]

Despite acceptance of this interventional therapy, a universal definition for fluid resuscitation does not exist. Byrne and Van Haren[10] define fluid resuscitation for sepsis as "the administration of fluid to correct sepsis-induced tissue hypoperfusion." This definition is aligned with the surviving sepsis guidelines.[3] The therapeutic effect of fluid resuscitation results from increasing venous return and CO.[3] Research and clinical evidence supporting the use of fluid resuscitation in patients with sepsis remains inconsistent and controversial. Avoiding aggressive and indiscriminate administration of fluids is important, as an overall positive fluid balance is associated with increased morbidity and mortality in sepsis.[12]

Because of the complexity of sepsis and septic shock, determining the best approach to fluid resuscitation is difficult, and goals depend on the patient's phase of illness.[12] Close monitoring of fluid administration is necessary because of the risk of edema from fluid overload.[13] Four phases of resuscitation were identified by Vincent and DeBacker[13] to guide fluid resuscitation: salvage (rescue) phase, optimization phase, stabilization phase, and deescalation phase.[13] Adequate hemodynamic support of patients in shock requires that resuscitation begin while the investigation of the cause is ongoing to prevent further organ dysfunction and failure.

In multiple studies of IV fluid resuscitation, using either goal-directed therapy or standard care, an average of more than 4 L of fluids was administered during the initial 6 hours of resuscitation, and in hours 6 to 72, the average was more than 8 L.[1] Recently, the safety of fluid resuscitation in patients with sepsis has been challenged, as prospective and observational data suggest improved patient outcomes with less fluid administration.,[10] The continuation of large-volume fluid administration beyond the initial period may be detrimental.[10,11] There is no prospective evidence demonstrating the benefit of fluid resuscitation as isolated therapy. There are significant concerns based on current research and clinical evidence that warrants research focused on the evaluation of alternative fluid strategies in the resuscitation phase of sepsis[10] (**Table 1**).

Endpoints for fluid resuscitation
There are a number of hemodynamic, oxygenation, and echocardiographic endpoints that have been proposed as goals for resuscitation in patients with sepsis and severe sepsis; however, some of these endpoints are controversial, difficult to define, and difficult to clinically assess.[7,13] The SSC guidelines recommend a CVP of 8 to 12 mm Hg (12–15 if mechanically ventilated), SVO2 greater than 70%, and urine output greater than 0.5 mL/kg per hour.[3] However, it is well established that there is no relationship between CVP and intravascular volume and no relationship between CVP and fluid responsiveness.[7] Further, a review of outcome data of patients enrolled in the

Table 1 Determining the best approach to fluid resuscitation is difficult and goals depend on the patient's phase of illness	
Phases of Resuscitation	**Goals**
Salvage/Rescue: fluid resuscitation	Blood pressure and cardiac output compatible with immediate survival; life-saving measures
Optimization; state of compensated shock: assess fluid responsiveness and need for administration	Adequate cellular oxygen availability; optimal cardiac output, venous oxygen saturation, lactate level
Stabilization: fluids administered to provide daily requirements and replace ongoing losses	Prevention of organ dysfunction and further complications
Deescalation: fluids deliberately removed from the patient and the goal is a negative fluid balance	Wean from ventilator support (if applicable); wean from vasoactive agents; achieve a negative fluid balance

Data from Refs.[10–12]

saving sepsis campaign found that attainment of CVP >8 and SVO2 greater than 70% did not influence survival in septic shock[7] (**Table 2**).

Fluid overload

Due to the pathogenesis of sepsis, patients who are septic are susceptible to fluid overload.[12] It was traditionally believed that approximately one-third of IV infused crystalloid volume remained intravascular; however, recent evidence suggests that this percentage is much lower with as little as 5% remaining in the intravascular space.[12] Fluid overload can lead to acute kidney injury as a result of increased venous congestion, interstitial edema, and extrarenal compression from increases in intra-abdominal pressure.[12] Large-volume resuscitation in patients with sepsis may worsen the hemodynamic derangements of sepsis from a pathophysiological standpoint.[7]

Fluid overload is a state of excess total body water caused by increased fluid administration and decreased renal elimination in critical illness.[7] Multiple clinical studies have found an association with positive fluid balance and increased mortality.[7,11,13] In patients with more severe sepsis, fluids alone will likely exacerbate the vasodilatory shock, and increase capillary leak and tissue edema.[7] Clinicians should be concerned about initiating additional fluids after the initial resuscitation because this may increase edema, especially to organs such as the liver and kidney.[11] With progressive capillary leak, these encapsulated organs are unable to compensate for the increased volume, resulting in severe interstitial edema that can compress vital blood flow. Thus, the use of vasopressors early on is important to maintain effective MAP necessary for adequate organ perfusion and to limit the formation of edema. The adverse effects of excessive fluid administration can lead to a positive fluid balance and the potential for patient harm, including death.[12,15]

Recommendations

In the recently published SSC 2016, the use of fluid resuscitation as the first hemodynamic intervention in shock is listed as a strong recommendation, but with low-quality evidence.[3] Fluid resuscitation was not investigated as an independent therapy, only in

Table 2 Goals for resuscitation in patients with sepsis and severe sepsis		
CVP	**SVO2**	**UO**
• No relationship between CVP and intravascular volume	• Patients who are septic usually have a normal or increased SVO2 caused by oxygen extraction	• May be a valuable marker of renal perfusion in hypovolemia
• No relationship between CVP and fluid responsiveness	• SVO2 >70% has been considered a diagnostic criterion for sepsis[9]	• In sepsis, UO is associated with acute kidney injury and oliguria that occurs in the presence of marked global renal hyperemia • Titration of fluids to UO may result in fluid overload
	• SVO2 >90% may be considered an independent predictor of mortality[9]	

Abbreviations: CVP, central venous pressure; SVO2, venous oxygen saturation; UO, urine output.
Data from Rhodes A, Evans LE, Alhazzani W, et al. Surviving sepsis campaign: international guidelines for management of sepsis and septic shock: 2016. Intensive Care Med 2017;43:304–77; and Marik PE. Early management of severe sepsis: concepts and controversies. Chest 2014;145(6):1407–18.

conjunction with antibiotics, vasopressors, and intensity of medical care. In the 3 recently published multisite RCTs, patients assigned EGDT received significantly more fluids than patients receiving standard care.[9] In these studies, patients receiving EGDT did not show improvement in mortality, instead it was associated with increased ICU admissions and use of ICU resources.[9] These studies did not support the systematic use of EGDT, which includes more aggressive fluid resuscitation. However, in all 3 RCTS, patients in both the study and the control groups received early IV fluid resuscitation and antibiotic administration.[4]

The current recommendations from the National Quality Forum and SSC 2016 include administration of IV crystalloid solution at 30 mL/kg and IV broad-spectrum antibiotics within 3 hours of diagnosis.[4] Fluid resuscitation is necessary at the early stages of septic shock to maintain hemodynamic stability. However, regarding fluid therapy, there exists a question regarding whether fluid administration should continue beyond that period.[11] The results of recent studies indicate that large-volume fluid resuscitation in patients with sepsis should be reconsidered. Further, health care providers should consider how much fluid is needed, the timing of fluid administration, and the parameters needed to maintain a safe, but adequate fluid balance.

Leisman and colleagues[4] conducted a study (n = 1866) to evaluate the association of IV fluid initiation within 30 minutes of severe sepsis or septic shock once it was identified in the emergency department on hospital mortality and length of stay. IV fluid resuscitation initiated at different times was also compared. In 64% of participants IV fluids were initiated within 30 minutes, and in 86% of participants IV antibiotics were given within 180 minutes. Statistical analysis using multivariate regression adjusting for age, hypotension, acute organ dysfunction, and emergency severity index score, revealed that initiation of IV fluids within 30 minutes was associated with lower mortality (odds ratio 0.63; 95% CI 0.46–0.86) and 12% shorter length of stay (hazard ratio 1.14; 95% CI 1.02–1.27). In secondary analysis, mortality increased with later fluid resuscitation initiation, 13.3% (<30 minutes) versus 16% (31–60 minutes) and 16.9% (61–180 minutes).[4] This study attempted to determine association of initiating IV fluid resuscitation within 30 minutes of severe sepsis or septic shock identification in the emergency room with in-hospital mortality controlling for demographic, acuity, and treatment factors. The investigators found that early initiation of IV fluids was associated with reduced mortality and length of stay. However, this study is limited given that it analyzed only the timing of the initiation of IV fluid resuscitation, not the volume administered or the time of completion.

Surviving sepsis campaign guidelines 2016 recommendations for fluid resuscitation
The SSC 2016 Guideline focuses on early management of patients with sepsis or septic shock.[3] This guideline panel was divided into 5 sections and an extensive search strategy ensued with GRADE methodology applied to selection of outcomes. Panel members discussed, deliberated, and presented their draft statements to panel members. The recommendations are as follows:

- Sepsis is considered a medical emergency and resuscitation should begin immediately.
- In resuscitation from sepsis-induced hyperperfusion at least 30 mL/kg of IV crystalloid fluid be given in the first 3 hours (strong recommendation; low quality of evidence).
- Following initial fluid resuscitation, additional fluids should be guided by reassessment of hemodynamic status (clinical examination and hemodynamics: blood pressure, oxygen saturation, respiratory rate, temperature, urine output) and invasive and noninvasive monitoring.

- Assess cardiac function.
- Use dynamic over static variables to predict fluid responsiveness where available (weak recommendation; low quality of evidence).
- Target MAP 65 mm Hg in patients with septic shock requiring vasopressors (strong recommendation; moderate quality of evidence).
- Guide resuscitation to normalize lactate in patients with elevated lactate levels as a marker of tissue hypoperfusion (weak recommendation/low quality of evidence).

Types of Fluids

Fluid therapy is best tailored to specific indications and aggressive fluid administration should be restricted only to the resuscitation phase of septic shock.[11] In addition, the components of select fluids may affect patient outcomes.

Crystalloids

Normal saline (NS) is not a true physiologic solution and its use in fluid resuscitation for septic shock is not supported.[12] This solution contains 154 mEq/L of sodium and 154 mEq/L of chloride and can produce a hyperchloremic metabolic acidosis and increased risk of death.[7] The supraphysiologic concentration of NS is associated with adverse effects on the renal, splanchnic, circulatory, pulmonary, and coagulation systems.

Balanced salt solutions (lactated Ringers, Hartmann, Plasmalyte 148) are the preferred resuscitation fluids in sepsis.[7] Balanced crystalloid solutions may be superior to saline in sepsis resuscitation.[12]

Colloids

Albumin: Current guidelines recommend consideration of albumin in patients who continue to require substantial amounts of crystalloid administration to maintain MAP. Although albumin has a number of theoretic benefits in patients with sepsis, including antioxidant and anti-inflammatory effects, and the ability to stabilize the glycocalyx, there is not sufficient research evidence to support the routine use of albumin in the initial resuscitation of patients with severe sepsis or septic shock.[12]

Hydroxyethyl starch solutions are associated with an increased risk of renal failure and death in sepsis and are therefore contraindicated[12] (**Table 3**).

IMPLICATIONS FOR FUTURE RESEARCH

To provide a definitive answer regarding the true effect of fluid administration in the resuscitation phase of sepsis, high-level evidence from RCTs that compare fluid resuscitation with no fluid resuscitation is needed.[10] The only current RCT of fluid resuscitation in sepsis is the FEAST (fluid expansion as supportive therapy) trial that included 3141 children with severe sepsis to receive fluid resuscitation with 40 mL/kg of NS or 4% albumin or no volume resuscitation.[10] However, this study was stopped early on because of harm demonstrating a 40% increase in mortality in both the volume resuscitation groups.[10] The interpretation of the findings of the FEAST study may be specific to the population noted for a high incidence of malaria, severe anemia, and acidosis.

More research is needed to determine the most appropriate fluid volume to be administered in patients with sepsis.[10,15] Although numerous studies reported increased mortality risk with increasing antibiotic delay, most of these studies do not take into account whether an appropriately timed fluid bolus was administered. The association of time to IV fluid resuscitation has been investigated less extensively

Table 3 Fluids			
Fluids	**Risks**	**Benefits**	**Recommendations**
Lactated Ringers; Hartmann, Plasmalyte		Less effect on acid-base equilibrium than 0.9% saline; this balanced solution more closely approximates that of plasma[12]	Intravenous solution of choice for fluid resuscitation in sepsis
Normal saline	Hyperchloremic metabolic acidosis Increased risk of death[12]		Use balanced solution as first choice
Hydroxyethyl starch (HES) solutions	Associated with increased mortality and a trend toward a higher need for renal replacement therapy[12]		Avoid use in critically ill patients with sepsis
Albumin		Antioxidant and anti-inflammatory effects	

Data from Loflin R, Winters ME. Fluid resuscitation in severe sepsis. Emerg Med Clin North Am 2017;35:59–74.

despite a consensus on hypoxemic or hypoperfusion mechanism of injury and disease progression in sepsis. Although several studies demonstrate mortality benefits for increased IV fluid administration within 3 hours, more comprehensive stratification of time to resuscitation is sparse in the literature.[4]

SUMMARY

Although fluid resuscitation remains the cornerstone of early and aggressive treatment of patients with severe sepsis and septic shock, fundamental questions remain regarding optimal fluid composition, volume, and rate of fluid administration in patients with sepsis.[11,12] Current research evidence regarding aggressive fluid administration beyond the resuscitation phase of shock challenges health care providers to reconsider the fluid regimen,[11,15] and consider the concomitant administration of vasopressors along with fluids in the salvage or rescue phase of septic shock.[3,12] The management of sepsis requires an integrated approach of fluid administration, infection control, appropriate antibiotics, and supportive care to maintain hemodynamic stability.[11] The use of large-volume fluid resuscitation in sepsis beyond the initial recommended period may be detrimental to patient survival.[11,15]

REFERENCES

1. Gauer RL. Early recognition and management of sepsis in adults: the first six hours. Am Fam Physician 2013;88(1):44–53.
2. Scott MC. Defining and diagnosing sepsis. Emerg Med Clin North Am 2017;35: 1–9.
3. Rhodes A, Evans LE, Alhazzani W, et al. Surviving sepsis campaign: international guidelines for management of sepsis and septic shock: 2016. Intensive Care Med 2017;43:304–7.

4. Leisman D, Wie B, Doerfler M, et al. Association of fluid resuscitation within 30 minutes of severe sepsis and septic shock recognition with reduced mortality and length of stay. Ann Emerg Med 2016;68(3):298–311.
5. Peterson LN, Chase K. Pitfalls in the treatment of sepsis. Emerg Med Clin N Am 2017;35:185–98.
6. Singer M, Deutschman CS, Seymour C, et al. The third international consensus definitions for sepsis and septic shock (Sepsis-3). JAMA 2016;315(8):801–10.
7. Marik PE. Early management of severe sepsis: concepts and controversies. Chest 2014;145(6):1407–18.
8. Rivers E, Nguyen B, Havstad S, et al. Early goal-directed therapy in the treatment of severe sepsis and septic shock. N Engl J Med 2001;345:1368–77.
9. Angus DC, Barnato AE, Bell D. A systematic review and meta-analysis of early goal directed therapy for septic shock: the ARISE, ProCESS, and ProMISe Investigators. Intensive Care Med 2015;41(9):1549–60.
10. Byrne L, Van Haren F. Fluid resuscitation in human sepsis: time to rewrite history? Am J Emerg Med 2017;7(1):1–8.
11. Hariyanto H, Yahya CQ, Widiastuti M, et al. Fluids and sepsis: changing the paradigm of fluid therapy: a case report. J Med Case Rep 2017;11(1):1–7.
12. Loflin R, Winters ME. Fluid resuscitation in severe sepsis. Emerg Med Clin N Am 2017;35:59–74.
13. Vincent JL, Debacker D. Circulatory shock. N Engl J Med 2013;369:1726–34.
14. Marik P, Bellomo R. A rational approach to fluid therapy in sepsis. Br J Anaesth 2016;116(3):339–49.
15. Boyd JH, Forbes J, Nakada T, et al. Fluid resuscitation in septic shock: a positive fluid balance and elevated central venous pressure are associated with increased mortality. Crit Care Med 2011;39(2):259–65.

Beyond the Intensive Care Unit
Posttraumatic Stress Disorder in Critically Ill Patients

Jennifer B. Martin, DNP, CRNA*, Jennifer E. Badeaux, DNP, CRNA

KEYWORDS

• Posttraumatic stress disorder • Sepsis • Anxiety • Critically ill • Intensive care

KEY POINTS

- Posttraumatic stress disorder after surviving an intensive care unit (ICU) stay has been identified in approximately 9% to 27% of patients, compared with 7% of the general US population.
- As a result of increasing ICU survival rates, new light has been shed on the emotional consequences of being critically ill for patients in the ICU.
- Timely interventions and treatment may reduce the incidence of physical and psychological comorbid conditions in ICU patients.
- For the ICU nurse, a better understanding of posttraumatic stress disorder for critically ill patients surviving an ICU stay may lead to improved patient outcomes.

INTRODUCTION

Progresses in medical care have made it possible for more patients in the intensive care unit (ICU) to survive critical illnesses and return to daily living after a traumatic health event. As a result of this shift in survival rates, a new light has been shed on the emotional consequences of surviving a critical illness in the ICU. Of patients surviving an ICU stay, posttraumatic stress disorder (PTSD) has been identified in approximately 9% to 27% compared with 7% of the general US population. Risk factors that are associated with the development of PTSD in ICU patients include mechanical ventilation, sedation, previous mental health issues, delusional memories, and agitation. These patients are more likely to experience negative physical and psychiatric health outcomes and a lower quality of life than are patients who survive the ICU

Disclosure Statement: The authors have nothing to disclose.
Nurse Anesthesia Program, Louisiana State University Health New Orleans, School of Nursing, 1900 Gravier Street, New Orleans, LA 70112, USA
* Corresponding author.
E-mail address: jmar19@lsuhsc.edu

Crit Care Nurs Clin N Am 30 (2018) 333–342
https://doi.org/10.1016/j.cnc.2018.05.001
0899-5885/18/© 2018 Elsevier Inc. All rights reserved.

without PTSD. ICU practitioners have an important role to play with early identification of patients experiencing signs and symptoms of this disorder. Timely interventions and treatment may reduce the incidence of physical and psychological comorbid conditions. Interventions available to ICU providers that may be able to reduce signs and symptoms of PTSD in patients include vigilant monitoring of medications, early and frequent mobilization, sleep scheduling, and proper pain management. The purpose of this article is to inform the bedside ICU practitioner of the risk factors, incidence, and innovative therapies regarding ICU-related PTSD. This knowledge is useful in caring for critically ill patients, especially those with sepsis and septic shock who require an increased length of stay in the ICU.

BACKGROUND

Each year in the United States, millions of patients (approximately 5 million) require specialized treatment in an ICU.[1] Critical illnesses are life-threatening and traumatic, and many patients recall extremely fear-provoking ICU stays.[2] Therefore, PTSD is of particular concern in this patient population. Several studies have been published regarding post-ICU PTSD. Research in the field focuses on longer term outcomes of ICU-treated patients, including mental health, health-related quality of life, and cognitive outcomes.[3–5] For the ICU bedside practitioner, caring for the emotional well-being of their patients is just as important as treating physical conditions and disease processes.

Prevalence and Incidence

Sepsis (ie, the presence of infection together with systemic manifestations of infection) and severe sepsis are important and alarming public health issues. Sepsis is a systemic, deleterious host response to infection that eventually transitions into severe sepsis, which is characterized by acute organ dysfunction secondary to documented or suspected infection. Severe sepsis can also place a patient in septic shock, which is defined as severe sepsis plus hypotension not reversed with fluid resuscitation. To be classified as having severe sepsis, the patient must exhibit symptoms of sepsis and symptoms of sepsis-induced organ dysfunction.[6]

The Society of Critical Care Medicine has estimated that each year approximately 5 million patients are admitted to an ICU in the United States.[1] Hospitalization rates due to sepsis as a principal diagnosis has increased more than twofold, from 11.6 to 24.0 per 10,000 population between 2001 and 2008.[6] Sepsis accounts for more than 751,000 cases and 215,000 deaths in the United States annually.[7] Sepsis treatment is expensive and frequently involves a prolonged stay in the ICU with complex therapies and high costs. The Agency for Healthcare Research and Quality lists sepsis as the most expensive condition treated in US hospitals, costing nearly $24 billion in 2013.[8] People with sepsis are 2 to 3 times more likely to be readmitted to the hospital compared with people with many other conditions, including heart failure, pneumonia, and chronic obstructive pulmonary disease.[9]

Readmissions due to sepsis are also more expensive than readmissions due to any of these other conditions. The ICU practitioner must be aware that, with increasing rates of hospitalization and ICU admissions related to sepsis, these patients are at potential risk for development of PTSD symptoms following their ICU stay. The length of stay for a patient in the ICU is among the most important concerns for health professionals. Several factors may affect the length of stay in an ICU: medical severity factors, psychosocial factors, and institutional factors. Moreover, there are also many methods and management strategies that can influence the length of stay; for example, a higher nurse-to-patient ratio results in a lower hospital length of stay for ICU patients. Length of stay is the primary factor for hospitalization cost; in fact, the cost of caring for patients in ICU in the United States has been estimated to account for 1% to 2% of the gross national product and 15% to 20% of United States hospital costs, which represents 38% of total US health care costs. Because of this, reducing the length of stay for patients should be the primary concern of health care professionals.[10]

Clinical Significance

Critical illnesses, and the extensive treatments needed to optimize function, can expose patients to extreme stressors. Examples of these stressors, which effect every physiologic system, include respiratory insufficiency, pain with procedures, release of inflammatory cytokines, strain on the hypothalamic-pituitary-adrenal axis, administration of numerous vasopressors for blood pressure control, and delirium with associated psychotic experiences. In addition to these stressors, ICU patients are dealing with a limited ability to communicate and reduced autonomy.[2]

Patients who survive severe sepsis may return to normal daily living after an ICU stay. However, some patients, especially those with preexisting chronic diseases, may have permanent organ damage. There is also some evidence that severe sepsis disrupts a patient's immune system, which will put a patient at higher risk for future infections. Studies have shown that people who have experienced sepsis have a higher risk of various medical conditions and death, even several years after the episode.[6] Therefore, patients experiencing long ICU stays due to sepsis and sepsis-related illness are at potentially higher risk for developing signs and symptoms of PTSD than patients in non-ICU settings.

Differential Diagnosis

The ICU practitioner must consider several diagnosis for the patient who exhibits signs and symptoms of disorientation. The practitioner has the difficult task of deciphering between symptoms to make the appropriate diagnosis. However, the identification of risk factors, prevention, and treatment of the different conditions remain similar (**Table 1**).

To help prevent any course of delirium or ICU psychosis, many ICUs are implementing preventative measures. These include instituting more liberal visiting policies, allowing periods for sleep, protecting the patient from unnecessary excitement, minimizing shift changes in the nursing staff caring for a patient, orienting the patient to date and time, reviewing all medical procedures, asking the patient to express any questions or concerns, obtaining information regarding religious and cultural beliefs, and attempting to coordinate lighting with the normal day–night cycle.[11,12]

POSTTRAUMATIC STRESS DISORDER

PTSD is a severe anxiety disorder that some people develop after experiencing or witnessing a life-threatening event, such as combat, a natural disaster, a car accident, or sexual assault. The disorder is characterized by reexperience of the traumatic event via flashbacks or nightmares, and by arousal of the autonomic nervous system, which can be manifested as difficulty sleeping, irritability, and exaggerated startle response.[13] An estimated 7% to 8% of Americans (approximately 24.4 million people) have PTSD at any given time. PTSD symptoms usually start soon after the traumatic event; however, some people do not experience symptoms of the disorder until

Table 1
Diagnosis to consider in intensive care unit patients

Condition	Definition	Incidence	Risk Factors or Causes	Treatment
Delirium	Definition: A state of severe confusion and rapid alterations in brain function Onset: sudden Signs and symptoms: hallucinations, delusions and hyperactivity Pathophysiology: a neurobehavioral syndrome caused by the transient disruption of normal neuronal activity secondary to systemic disturbances	A meta-analysis of 42 studies and 16,595 critically ill subjects showed an occurrence rate of delirium of 31.8%	Causes: head injury, drug use or withdrawal, poisonings, brain tumors, infections, metabolic disturbances, or as a result of preexisting mental illness	Prognosis and treatment: depends on the underlying cause of the condition
Psychosis	Definition: a disorder in which patients in an ICU or a similar setting display a cluster of serious psychiatric symptoms (ie, ICU syndrome) Onset: within 1 to 5 days of ICU stay Signs and symptoms: a cluster of psychiatric symptoms, including but not limited to anxiety, restlessness, hallucinations, nightmares, and paranoia Pathophysiology: ICU psychosis is also a form of delirium or acute brain failure in which the pathogenetic mechanisms are not well-understood	Estimates are that 1 in every 3 patients who spend more than 5 days in an ICU experiences some form of psychotic reaction Non-ICU departments should be aware of this phenomenon because increasing numbers of ICU patients are being transferred out of the ICU more rapidly than in years past	While in the ICU, symptoms often vanish with the coming of morning or the arrival of some sleep Symptoms may linger throughout the day, with agitation worsening at night, (ie, sundowning) Additional triggers, such as environmental (sensory and sleep deprivation), along with medical causes (pain, infection, analgesia)	Prognosis: usually resolves completely when the patient leaves the ICU Treatment: the primary goal is to correct any imbalance, restore the patient's health, and return the patient to normal activities as quickly as possible

Data *from* Refs.[11–13]

months or years later. The disorder is diagnosed if the symptoms persist longer than 4 weeks, cause great distress, or interfere with work or home life. There are 4 types of symptoms of PTSD; however, notably, each person experiences symptoms in their own way[14]:

1. Reliving the event: The person may have bad memories or nightmares. This is also known as a flashback.
2. Avoiding situations: The person will try to avoid situations or people that trigger memories of the traumatic event.
3. Having more negative beliefs and feelings: The way a person thinks about themselves and others may change because of the trauma. They may feel guilt or shame, or lose interest in activities they used to enjoy. Some patients report feeling numb to the world.
4. Hyperarousal: The person may be jittery, or always alert and on the lookout for danger. They may also experience trouble concentrating or sleeping.[13]

Statistics and Information of the General Population

The Department of Veteran Affairs,[14] National Institutes of Health,[15] and the Sidran Institute[16] confirm that the societal and economic burden of PTSD is extremely heavy. Some important truths regarding PTSD include

- The annual societal cost of anxiety disorders is estimated to be approximately $42 billion.
- Patients diagnosed with PTSD have among the highest usage rates of health care services.
- PTSD was first recognized as a disorder with specific symptoms that could be reliably diagnosed in 1980. It was then added to the American Psychiatric Association's *Diagnostic and Statistical Manual of Mental Disorders*.[13]
- PTSD is recognized as a psychobiological mental disorder affecting survivors of all forms of traumatic experiences, including combat, terror attacks, natural disasters, serious accidents, assault, or abuse, and (most recently discovered) ICU stays.
- PTSD is associated with changes in the function and structure of the brain. These changes provide clues to the origins, treatment, and prevention of PTSD.
- Approximately half of all outpatient mental health patients are diagnosed with PTSD.
- According to Veterans Administration, experts estimate that up to 20% of Operation Enduring Freedom and Operation Iraqi Freedom veterans, up to 10% of Gulf War veterans, and up to 30% of Vietnam War veterans have experienced PTSD.

What is Intensive Care Unit–Related Posttraumatic Stress Disorder?

The Society of Critical Care Medicine[1] has estimated that each year 5 million patients in the United States will be admitted to an ICU. Critically ill patients are receiving innovative treatments and, as a result, survival rates have improved. This increasing number of survivors are discharged home or to a long-term care facility to make a meaningful recovery. This change in survival has led to an increased attention on the emotional and physical consequences of these lifesaving interventions during times of critical illness.[17]

Incidence in Intensive Care Unit Patients and Survivors

The stressful experience of a life-threatening illness or trauma can place ICU patients at a particularly higher risk for PTSD compared with other patients. This is due in part to the treatments and interventions received in the ICU.[17] These critically ill patients may have a more complicated recovery than do other patients because PTSD is associated with higher rates of coronary heart disease, chronic pain, gastrointestinal disorders, arthritis, and decreased quality of life.[18–21]

Researchers at Johns Hopkins University School of Medicine conducted a systematic review and discovered the prevalence of PTSD ranged from 10% to 60%. Forty studies were included in the review, consisting of 36 unique subject cohorts with a total of more than 3000 subjects who survived a critical illness requiring an ICU stay. Exclusion criteria consisted of patients who had suffered a trauma because those patients' cognitive and psychological outcomes may be affected by the injury itself, rather than the critical illness or the ICU stay.

To determine a more decisive estimate of PTSD prevalence, the researchers then conducted a meta-analysis of a subset of the 40 studies found through a systematic review. They selected 6 studies that used a PTSD measurement tool called the Impact of Event Scale between 1 and 6 months after ICU discharge, with a total of approximately 450 subjects. From these data, they established that 1 in 4 subjects had symptoms of PTSD. The researchers repeated the same meta-analysis for studies that looked at subjects 7 to 12 months after an ICU stay and found that 1 in 5 subjects had PTSD.[22]

Nursing Implications for Recognizing and Managing Risk Factors

Some common risk factors for PTSD discovered through research are a previous history and diagnosis of a psychological problem, such as anxiety or depression. Another risk factor for development of ICU-related PTSD is a patient receiving large amounts of sedation medication while in the ICU. In addition, patients experiencing frightening memories of the ICU have a higher risk of PTSD. Symptoms are found to occur across a wide variety of patients, regardless of their age, diagnosis, severity of illness, or length of stay.[22] However, Davydow and colleagues[23] (2008) concluded that pretrauma psychopathology, female sex, and younger age emerged as general risk factors for PTSD. The factors that ICU practitioners must be aware of when caring for patients at risk for developing ICU-related PTSD follow.

PERSONAL FACTORS

- Prior psychopathology, such as anxiety and depressive disorders before ICU admission.[23]
- Female patients younger than 65 years are at greater risk than are male patients or older patients for ICU-related PTSD.[24–26]

INTENSIVE CARE UNIT FACTORS

The ICU is an environment conducive for development of ICU-related PTSD due to multiple factors. These include but are not limited to use of specific medications, such as vasopressors and sedatives; use of mechanical ventilation; delusional memories of the ICU; and agitation. Nurses may be better prepared to identify and potentially diminish some of the risk factors if made aware while providing care for critically ill patients.

Vasopressors

- Vasopressors used to combat hypotension (phenylephrine and norepinephrine) and inotropes (dopamine and dobutamine), were correlated with anxiety in a prospective cohort study 3 of 100 mixed diagnosis ICU subjects.[26]

- Use of vasopressors for an extended time creates a chronic stress state.[26]
- Female patients who receive beta-antagonists (metoprolol) following cardiac surgery have a lower incidence of PTSD signs and symptoms with fewer traumatic memories 6 months after surgery compared with the control group not receiving metoprolol.[27]

Sedation

- Use of benzodiazepines and duration of sedation are associated with signs and symptoms of PTSD.[28]
- Benzodiazepines have an amnesic effect and amnesia has been positively correlated with higher levels of PTSD signs and symptoms.[29]
- The relationship between the use of spontaneous awakening trials and a reduction in PTSD signs and symptoms has not been validated.[30]
- Lighter levels of sedation may be more beneficial than a focus on the more time-consuming spontaneous awakening trial.[30]

Mechanical Ventilation

- An association between mechanical ventilation and signs and symptoms of PTSD in mixed-diagnosis ICU patients exists according to the evidence.[17,23,28]
- Longer duration of mechanical ventilation has been associated with increased risk for PTSD in patients who survive acute lung injury or acute respiratory distress syndrome.[23]
- The ICU practitioner may have an opportunity to reduce risk for PTSD in ICU patients by advocating for interventions that promote earlier extubation, such as spontaneous breathing trials, lighter levels of sedation, and early mobilization.

Delusional Memories

- Delusional memories in the ICU setting are memories of frightening perceptual experiences patients had while critically ill.[31]
- The association between PTSD, delusional memories, and delirium is mixed. Delusional memories are associated with the development of PTSD and are more likely to be retained over time than factual memories.[31]
- Currently, no association between delirium and increased risk for PTSD has been reported.[22,25]

Agitation

- Agitation is often first managed with medications causing sedation; however, if sedation is contraindicated, physical restraints are used. Episodes of agitation and use of restraints are associated with PTSD.[23]
- ICU practitioners must recognize agitation in patients and quickly define the underlying cause (pain, delirium, and hypoxemia) before treating patients with benzodiazepines. Nonbenzodiazepines may be more helpful than benzodiazepines for treatment of agitation in patients who are not experiencing alcohol withdrawal.[30]
- Patients experiencing stress, fear, loss of control, and an inability to express their wishes are at a higher risk for PTSD than are patients not experiencing these conditions.[28]

Severity of Illness and Length of Intensive Care Unit Stay

- Current research is not conclusive regarding these 2 factors that may be major contributors to the development of PTSD in ICU patients.

- Length of stay and severity of illness, as measured by using the Acute Physiology and Chronic Health Evaluation II, have not been consistently associated with the development of PTSD in critically ill patients.[24,26]

INTERVENTIONS TO REDUCE POSTTRAUMATIC STRESS DISORDER SYMPTOMS

Prevention methods have been revealed though research, although many other studies need to be done to expand this knowledge base. Based on results of a systematic review on the effects of nonpharmacological interventions and ICU-related stress, the most significant difference in stress levels were found with implementation of an ICU diary.[32] This is a notebook that allows clinicians and family members to write daily messages about what is happening to the patient. Diary writing may assist patients with processing their experience and formulate more accurate memories of their time in the ICU. It is thought that ICU diaries may lessen the impact of delusional memories, which are associated with post-ICU PTSD by strengthening factual memories. Although very few institutions in the United States are using ICU diaries, they are commonly used in critical care units throughout Europe.[31]

Other interventions used to reduce patient distress in the ICU setting that can used on a daily basis by the ICU care team include playing music and nature sounds, family-delivered massage and reflexology, and collaborative songwriting therapy. These interventions are generally low-risk to the patient and easy to implement by the ICU practitioner. Although more follow-up studies need to be done to demonstrate the long-term effects of these interventions, the decrease in acute anxiety and stress levels was adequately proven.[31]

SUMMARY

The ICU is a chaotic setting for patients and sometimes can cause extreme traumatic memories, leading to the development of PTSD. ICU practitioners caring for the growing population of ICU survivors should be aware of PTSD risk factors and monitor patients' needs for early intervention. Regularly scheduled patient assessment for the presence of risk factors during routine physical assessment and medication review may allow ICU nurses to intervene directly or advocate for treatments. In addition, collaboration is needed between intensivists, primary care physicians, and psychiatrists to ensure prompt, comprehensive evaluations and treatment of patients experiencing traumatic stays in the ICU.

ACKNOWLEDGMENTS

Cade T. Martin significantly contributed to the writing and research of this article.

REFERENCES

1. Society of Critical Care Medicine. Critical care statistics. Available at: http://www.sccm.org/Communications/Pages/CriticalCareStats.aspx. Accessed December 6, 2017.
2. Jones C, Griffiths RD, Humphris G. Disturbed memory and amnesia related to intensive care. Memory 2000;8:79–94.
3. Broomhead LR, Brett SJ. Clinical review: intensive care follow-up - what has it told us? Crit Care 2002;6:411–7.
4. Dowdy DW, Eid MP, Sedrakyan A, et al. Quality of life in adult survivors of critical illness: a systematic review of the literature. Intensive Care Med 2005;31:611–20.

5. Hopkins RO, Jackson JC. Long-term neurocognitive function after critical illness. Chest 2006;130:869–78.
6. Hall MJ, Williams SN, DeFrances CJ, et al. Inpatient care for septicemia or sepsis: a challenge for patients and hospitals. NCHS Data Brief 2011;62:1–8.
7. Angus DC, Linde-Zwirble WT, Lidicker J, et al. Epidemiology of severe sepsis in the United States: analysis of incidence, outcome, and associated costs of care. Crit Care Med 2001;29:1303–10.
8. Agency for Healthcare Research and Quality Healthcare Cost and Utilization Project Statistical Brief No. 204; 2016. National inpatient hospital costs: the most expensive conditions by payer, 2013.
9. Mayr FB, Talisa VB, Balakumar V, et al. Proportion and cost of unplanned 30-day readmissions after sepsis compared with other medical conditions. JAMA 2017;317(5):530–1. Available at: https://jamanetwork.com/journals/jama/fullarticle/2598785.
10. Gonzalez JM. National Health Care Expenses in the U.S. Civilian Noninstitutionalized Population, 2011. MEPS Statistical Brief No. 425. Rockville (MD): Agency for Healthcare Research and Quality; 2013. Available at: http://meps.ahrq.gov/data_files/publications/st425/stat425.pdf. Accessed January 28, 2018.
11. Maldonado JR. Acute brain failure: pathophysiology, diagnosis, management, and sequelae of delirium. Crit Care Clin 2017;33:461–519.
12. Salluh JIF, Wang H, Schneider EB, et al. Outcome of delirium in critically ill patients: systematic review and meta-analysis. BMJ 2015;350:h2538.
13. American Psychiatric Association. Diagnostic and statistical manual of mental disorders. 5th edition. Washington, DC: American Psychiatric Publishing; 2013.
14. U.S. Department of Veterans Affairs. PTSD: National Center for PTSD. Available at: https://www.ptsd.va.gov/professional/PTSD-overview/index.asp. Accessed January 17, 2018.
15. National Institutes of Health: fighting PTSD. Available at: https://fightingptsd.wordpress.com/tag/national-institutes-of-health/. Accessed December 10, 2017.
16. Sidran Institute: Traumatic Stress Education & Advocacy. Available at: https://www.sidran.org/resources/for-survivors-and-loved-ones/post-traumatic-stress-disorder-fact-sheet-2/. Accessed January 7, 2018.
17. Wade DM, Howell DC, Weinman JA, et al. Investigating risk factors for psychological morbidity three months after intensive care: a prospective cohort study. Crit Care 2012;16(5):R192.
18. Edmondson D, Kronish IM, Shaffer JA, et al. Posttraumatic stress disorder and risk for coronary heart disease: a meta-analytic review. Am Heart J 2013;166(5):806–14.
19. Sareen J, Cox BJ, Stein M, et al. Physical and mental comorbidity, disability, and suicidal behavior associated with posttraumatic stress disorder in a large community sample. Psychosom Med 2007;69(3):242–8.
20. Qureshi SU, Pyne JM, Magruder KM, et al. The link between post traumatic stress disorder and physical comorbidities: a systematic review. Psychiatr Q 2009;80(2):87–97.
21. Jackson JC, Mitchell N, Hopkins RO. Cognitive functioning, mental health, and quality of life in ICU survivors: an overview. Crit Care Clin 2011;25(3):615–28.
22. Bienvenu J, Colantuoni E, Mendez-Tellez PA, et al. Co-occurrence of and remission from general anxiety, depression, and posttraumatic stress disorder symptoms after acute lung injury. Crit Care Med 2015;43(3):642.
23. Davydow DS, Gifford JM, Desai SV, et al. Posttraumatic stress disorder in general intensive care unit survivors: a systematic review. Gen Hosp Psychiatry 2008;30(5):421–34.

24. Wallen K, Chaboyer W, Thalib L, et al. Symptoms of acute posttraumatic stress disorder after intensive care. Am J Crit Care 2008;17(6):534–41.

25. Girard T, Shintani A, Jackson J, et al. Risk factors for post-traumatic stress disorder symptoms following critical illness requiring mechanical ventilation: a prospective cohort study. Crit Care 2007;11(1):R28.

26. Ratzer M, Romano E, Elklit A. Posttraumatic stress disorder in patients following intensive care unit treatment: a review of studies regarding prevalence and risk factors. J Trauma Treat 2014;3(190):1–15.

27. Krauseneck T, Padberg F, Roozendaal B, et al. A beta-adrenergic antagonist reduces traumatic memories and PTSD symptoms in female but not in male patients after cardiac surgery. Psychol Med 2010;40(5):861–9.

28. Wade D, Hardy R, Howell D, et al. Identifying clinical and acute psychological risk factors for PTSD after critical care: a systematic review. Minerva Anestesiol 2013; 79(8):944–63.

29. Granja C, Gomes E, Amaro A, et al. Understanding posttraumatic stress disorder-related symptoms after critical care: the early illness amnesia hypothesis. Crit Care Med 2008;36(10):2801–9.

30. Barr J, Fraser GL, Puntillo K, et al. Clinical practice guidelines for the management of pain, agitation, and delirium in adult patients in the intensive care unit. Crit Care Med 2013;41(1):263–306.

31. Jones C, Backman C, Capuzz o M, et al. Intensive care diaries reduce new-onset post traumatic stress disorder following critical illness: a randomised, controlled trial. Crit Care 2010;14:R168.

32. Wade DM, Moon Z, Windgassen SS, et al. Non-pharmacological interventions to reduce ICU-related psychological distress: a systematic review. Minerva Anestesiol 2016;82(4):465–78.

Emerging Adjunctive Approach for the Treatment of Sepsis: Vitamin C and Thiamine

Jennifer E. Badeaux, DNP, CRNA,
Jennifer B. Martin, DNP, CRNA*

KEYWORDS

- Sepsis • Septic shock • Adjuvant treatment • Vitamin C • Thiamine

KEY POINTS

- Sepsis is defined as "life-threatening organ dysfunction caused by a dysregulated host response to infection."
- Sepsis affects approximately 1.5 million people each year in the United States.
- Sepsis is the most expensive condition being treated in US hospitals, costing more than $24 billion in 2014.
- Vitamin C has been hypothesized to be a cost-effective and novel adjuvant therapy that can be used to ameliorate the effects of inflammation and oxidative stress in sepsis.

INTRODUCTION

Sepsis is a clinical condition that remains highly lethal. It is most often seen in critically ill patients and trauma victims. Sepsis and septic shock is a systemic and dysregulated inflammatory response to infection that can lead to hemodynamic instability, multiple organ dysfunction syndrome, and death.

In the late 1970s, it was estimated that 164,000 cases of sepsis occurred in the United States each year.[1] Since the 1970s, it is reported that rates of sepsis globally have increased.[2–4]

Today, according to the Centers for Disease Control and Prevention (CDC) 2017[5]

- More than 1.5 million people get sepsis each year in the United States
- About 250,000 Americans die from sepsis each year
- One in three patients who die in a hospital has sepsis
- A CDC evaluation found 7 in 10 patients with sepsis had recently used health care services or had chronic diseases requiring frequent medical care

Disclosure: The authors have nothing to disclose.
Nurse Anesthesia Program, School of Nursing, Louisiana State University Health New Orleans, 1900 Gravier Street, New Orleans, LA 70112, USA
* Corresponding author.
E-mail address: jmar19@lsuhsc.edu

The incidence of sepsis is rising for several different reasons: the aging population, the increase in the use of invasive and immunosuppressive treatments in the older patient, and the increase in education and awareness campaigns for sepsis.[1,6–8] Neonates, the elderly, and those with weakened immune systems are most likely to get sepsis. Patients aged 65 years or older account for the majority (60%–85%) of all incidence of sepsis.[1] It is also highly likely that the incidence of sepsis will continue to increase in the future because of the aging population.[1,7] Unfortunately, treatment for sepsis is significantly challenging and is becoming even more so as drug-resistant infections become more widespread. According to the Agency for Healthcare Research and Quality, sepsis is the most expensive condition being treated in US hospitals, costing more than $24 billion in 2014.[9]

Sepsis and Septic Shock Defined

In 2016, a new definition of sepsis, Sepsis-3, was published in The Journal of the American Medical Association (JAMA). This published definition presented a drastic change from the prior sepsis definitions published in 1991 (Sepsis-1) and 2001 (Sepsis-2). The Sepsis-3 consensus definition makes no division between sepsis and the condition described by Sepsis-2 as severe sepsis (that is, sepsis with acute organ dysfunction).[10] According to the Sepsis-3 consensus, sepsis and severe sepsis are synonymous terms; therefore, currently there are only sepsis and septic shock.[10] The new classifications define sepsis as life-threatening organ dysfunction due to a dysregulated host response to infection. Septic shock is currently defined as a subset of sepsis in which particularly profound circulatory, cellular, and metabolic abnormalities substantially increase mortality.[10] The new definitions for sepsis and septic shock reveal significant advances made in the pathophysiology, management, and epidemiology of sepsis. These concise definitions describe the life-threatening conditions more precisely and are aimed at achieving greater precision and consistency in how sepsis is diagnosed, reported, and treated.[10]

Pathophysiology

The normal host response to infection is a multifaceted process that confines and controls a bacterial invasion as the injured tissue begins to heal.[11] Sepsis results when the response to the infection becomes systemic and affects normal tissues and organ systems distant from the initial injury or infection.[11] Patients then present an immune response that starts the activation of biochemical cytokines and mediators associated with an inflammatory response. Proinflammatory and antiinflammatory cytokines released during the inflammatory response directly influence the endothelium, cardiovascular, hemodynamic, and coagulation mechanisms.[11] It is known that widespread distribution of proinflammatory mediators play an important role in the pathogenesis and high morbidity and mortality associated with sepsis. The immune system goes into overdrive, overwhelming normal processes in the blood. Increased capillary permeability and vasodilation interrupt the body's ability to provide adequate perfusion, oxygen, and nutrients to the tissues and cells. The result is that small blood clots form, blocking blood flow to vital organs, which often lead to complete organ failure.[11] In addition to the imbalance of the inflammatory response, major vitamins are overwhelmingly consumed. An excessive inflammatory response indeed enhances metabolic turnover of vitamin C. As a result, patients with severe sepsis often have very low plasma vitamin C levels that sometimes enter the "scurvy" zone.[11]

Current Treatment

The new Surviving Sepsis Guidelines were released in January 2017. **Table 1** shows the updates to the 2012 guidelines. Following the Emmanuel Rivers' study in 2001, the 2012 sepsis criteria maintained the model of "early goal-directed therapy" (EGDT) as a guiding principle. This became the standard of care until the new guidelines were released in 2017.[12] The 2017 Surviving Sepsis Guidelines now reflect the results of the PROCESS, PROMISE, and ARISE trials—3 large multicenter studies demonstrating no significant difference in the primary outcome of mortality between EGDT and usual care.[13–15]

Table 1
Surviving sepsis campaign changes

Surviving Sepsis Campaign Updates- 2016		
Sepsis Definition	*Sepsis*: Life-threatening organ dysfunction caused by dysregulated host response to infection *Septic Shock*: Subset of sepsis with circulatory and cellular/metabolic dysfunction associated with higher risk of mortality	
Initial Resuscitation Parameters	During first 6 h the treatment protocol should include the following: • CVP 8–12 mm Hg • MAP ≥65 mm Hg • Urine output ≥0.5 mL/kg/h • $Scvo_2$ ≥70% (insert early) • normalize elevated lactate levels and use as a marker of tissue perfusion	
Fluid Therapy	At least 30 mL/kg of IV crystalloid fluid be given within the first 3 h Following initial fluid resuscitation, additional fluids should be guided by frequent reassessment of hemodynamic status Use albumin in addition to crystalloids when patients require substantial amounts of crystalloids	
Vasopressors	Use norepinephrine as the first-choice vasopressor Add either vasopressin (up to 0.03 U/min) or epinephrine to norepinephrine with the intent of raising MAP to target, or add vasopressin (up to 0.03 U/min) to decrease norepinephrine dosage	
Steroids	Only use IV hydrocortisone at a dose of 200 mg/d if septic shock refractory to adequate fluid and vasopressors	
Antibiotics	Initiate IV antimicrobials after recognition and within 1 h for both sepsis and septic shock Administer an empirical combination therapy (using at least 2 antibiotics of different antimicrobial classes) aimed at the most likely bacterial pathogen(s) for the initial management of septic shock Use procalcitonin levels to assess deescalation of antimicrobial therapy	
Source Control	Appropriate intervention should be implemented as soon as medically and logistically practical after the anatomic diagnosis of infection is made	
Ventilator	Sepsis-induced ARDS • Higher PEEP and lower tidal volumes • Prone over supine position • Pao_2/Fio_2 ratio <150 • NO HFOV	Sepsis-induced respiratory failure Without ARDS • Lower tidal volumes over higher tidal volumes

Abbreviations: ARDS, acute respiratory distress syndrome; CVP, central venous pressure; HFOV, high-frequency oscillation ventilation; IV, intravenous; MAP, mean arterial pressure; PEEP, positive end-expiratory pressure.

Data from Rhodes A, Evans LE, Alhazzani W, et al. Surviving sepsis campaign: international guidelines for management of sepsis and septic shock. Crit Care Med 2017;43(3):304–77.

The current sepsis treatment recommended by the Surviving Sepsis Campaign is directed at timely identification and treatment of infection through antibiotic administration, early source control, hemodynamic stability through fluid resuscitation, and use of vasopressors if necessary.[16] Although shock may be prevented by these supportive treatments, patients with severe sepsis can still die of multisystem organ failure even with adequate perfusion and cardiac output.[17] Much of the published research suggests that deaths in septic patients are often attributable to the microvascular dysfunction due to inflammation.[18] However, current sepsis treatment as described earlier does not target the inflammatory and oxidative stress caused by sepsis. In fact, the current standard therapies can potentially increase inflammation and cause further damage through the bactericidal effects of antibiotic administration.[19] Clearly, there is a need for new, targeted adjuvant therapies that reverse the inflammatory and oxidative stress present in septic patients; however, search for an effective targeted therapy continues to challenge researchers (see **Table 1**).

Finding/In Search of a Cure for Sepsis

A definitive cure for sepsis has puzzled physicians and scientists since the origination of contemporary medicine. Over the years scientists have made considerable progress in the diagnosis and management of sepsis, but there remains no definite treatment of this deadly condition.[9] There was a promising breakthrough in 2001 when the Food and Drug Administration approved the recombinant activated protein C, drotrecogin alfa (Xigris), for the treatment of sepsis. Unfortunately, drotrecogin alfa (Xigris) had to be pulled from the market in 2011 when a large postmarketing study failed to show significant efficacy.[20] Additional treatments such as hemofiltration have shown some promise but remain mostly experimental and are not in wide use.[9] Over the past 30 years, more than 100 phase 2 and phase 3 clinical trials have been done to test various novel pharmacologic agents and therapeutic interventions in an effort to improve the outcome of patients with severe sepsis and septic shock.[21] These trails ultimately failed to produce a novel pharmacologic agent that improved the outcome of sepsis.[12]

Treatment Options in Septic Patients: Vitamin C and Thiamine

Vitamin C and thiamine are both water-soluble vitamins that are involved in multiple biosynthetic and metabolic processes. Vitamin C dissociates at physiologic pH to form ascorbate, the redox state of the vitamin, which is found most abundantly in cells. Thiamine exists in the body in different forms but is essential for producing energy from glucose.[21]

Vitamin C

In healthy fasting humans, circulating levels of vitamin C are typically in the range of 50 to 70 µmol/L. Levels less than 25 µmol/L reflect marginal deficiency (hypovitaminosis C). Severe or scurvylike vitamin C deficiency is present when levels decrease below 10 µmol/L.[22] In the critical care setting, vitamin C is particularly known for its strong immunomodulation and antioxidant activity. An excessive inflammatory response enhances metabolic turnover of vitamin C. As such, vitamin C is promoted as adjuvant therapy in conditions characterized by excessive oxidative stress or crippled immunity, such as ischemia-reperfusion disorders, trauma, and various inflammatory disease processes.[23] Vitamin C is also required for the synthesis of catecholamines and cortisol, so deficiency causes failure of the sympathetic nervous system as well. It is well known that vitamins become depleted during sepsis and vitamin C levels consistently decrease, sometimes dropping below the level of detection. The intestinal absorption of vitamin C is limited, so the only way to replete vitamin C in patients with increased metabolic consumption of vitamin C in critical illness is to infuse it intravenously (IV).

Thiamine

Thiamine deficiency is also prevalent in patients with septic shock, with rates ranging from 20% to 70% depending on the cutoff value used to define the presence of thiamine deficiency.[24] Thiamine is a water soluble vitamin that is necessary in cellular metabolism. The lack of thiamine, therefore, can be life threatening.[24] In a prospective, observational study by Donnino and colleagues,[25] the relationship between thiamine levels and lactic acidosis in 30 septic shock patients was researched. The investigator found no correlation between these 2 variables. The investigator then excluded patients with abnormal liver function tests and a significant negative correlation between thiamine concentrations and lactic acidosis ($P = .01$). This shows a possible association between thiamine levels and lactic acidosis in septic shock patients with normal liver function.[25] A randomized control trial published by the same investigators found that patients given thiamine had lower lactate concentrations at 24 hours compared with the patients who were not administered thiamine. In addition, only 7% of patients given IV thiamine had lactate concentration higher than or equal to 4 mmol/L compared with 38% of patients who did not receive IV thiamine. The investigators also concluded that the in-hospital mortality was higher in the patients who did not receive the IV thiamine, but it was not statistically significant (46% vs. 13%, $P = .1$). However, the investigators observed a statistically significant difference in time to death in favor of the patients who received thiamine.[26] All these results suggest that the administration of thiamine is advantageous in septic shock patients with severe thiamine deficiency (thiamine level ≤7 nmol/L).[26]

Recent clinical and experimental data are showing promising evidence for the use of vitamin C and thiamine as adjuvants to treat sepsis and septic shock. **Table 2** compares recent studies using vitamin C and thiamine in patients with sepsis.[21,27–30] The most recently published and controversial study was conducted by Marik and colleagues.[21] The retrospective study looked at the role of vitamin C, thiamine, and hydrocortisone in patients with sepsis. The findings of the study were that early treatment with vitamin C, thiamine, and hydrocortisone produces a reduction of mortality in patients with severe sepsis and septic shock. This is one study and is limited by its single-centered design, with small sample size, but had statistically significant results with well-matched controls.

It is unclear exactly how important vitamin deficiencies may be to the pathogenesis of sepsis. However, it is not difficult to imagine that several different vitamin deficiencies could synergize to accompany organ failure.

DISCUSSION

Sepsis is a serious life-threatening condition with high morbidity and mortality rates. There have been several investigations into potential therapies for sepsis using targeted adjuvant therapies; however, many of them have failed to improve clinical outcomes in the treatment of sepsis.

Evidence is emerging that parenteral administration of high-dose vitamin C and thiamine may be a beneficial adjuvant therapy of severe sepsis and septic shock. Despite modern practices in critical care medicine, sepsis and severe sepsis remain a leading cause of morbidity and mortality in the critical care unit.

Patients with sepsis are perpetually deficient in vitamin C and frequently deficient in thiamine. Vitamin C is suggested to be a cost-effective and novel adjuvant therapy that

Table 2
Comparison of recent studies using vitamin C and thiamine in patients with sepsis

Study	Design	N	Dose of Vitamin C (RDA 60 mg/d)	Findings	Mortality Benefit
Marik et al,[21] 2017	Single-center retrospective before-after	47	1.5 g IV every 6 h	Early treatment with vitamin C, thiamine, and hydrocortisone saw a reduction of mortality in patients with severe sepsis and septic shock	Control: 40.4% mortality Treatment: 8.5% mortality $P<.001$
Fowler et al,[27] 2014	Single-center randomized double-blind placebo controlled trial	24	50 mg/kg or 200 mg/kg IV infusion every 24 h	Patients receiving vitamin C exhibited less inflammation and prompt reduction of organ failure	Study not powered to assess mortality
Natarajan et al,[28] 2014	Single-center retrospective randomized	24	50 mg/kg or 200 mg/kg IV infusion every 24 h	Decrease in biomarkers of sepsis (cfDNA and mtDNA) and decrease in RDW	Study not powered to assess mortality
Zabet et al,[29] 2016	Single-center double-blinded randomized controlled trial	28	25 mg/kg IV every 6 h	Reduction of norepinephrine requirement and decreased mortality in treatment with vitamin C	Control: 64.28% mortality Treatment:14.28% mortality $P = .009$
Tanaka et al,[30] 2000	Single-center prospective randomized study	37	66 mg/kg IV based off body surface area burned and urine output	Reduction of resuscitation fluid volume requirements, body weight gain, wound edema, and respiratory dysfunction	Control: 38.9% mortality Treatment: 47.3% mortality $P = .97$

Abbreviations: cfDNA, cell-free DNA; mtDNA, mitochondrial DNA; N, number; RDA, recommended dietary allowance; RDW, red cell distribution width.

can be used to improve the effects of inflammation and oxidative stress in sepsis. Deficiencies in vitamin C and thiamine might explain many of the abnormalities seen in sepsis. Vitamin C and thiamine have an outstanding track record of safety, which is proved over decades of experimentation and clinical experience. Five recent studies have suggested benefit from vitamin C or thiamine in critically ill patients, with no evidence of toxicity.[21,27–30] A recent before-after study found a substantial mortality benefit from the combination of stress-dose steroid, IV vitamin C, and IV thiamine. This study is not an RTC so additional research is warranted. However, it is a reasonable intervention given the excellent safety profile of these agents.[21]

According to this article, the following recommendations can be made:

- A baseline vitamin C concentration must be obtained in all patients and vitamin C should be given if levels are less than 25 μmol/L.
- In patients not treated with CRRT, 3 to 6 g vitamin C daily should be supplemented as long as vasopressor treatment is required. If CRRT is running, this dose can be temporarily increased to 12 g/d.
- The addition of low-dose hydrocortisone (50 mg every 6h), thiamine (200 mg every 12h), and high-dose vitamin C (1.5 g every 6h) to the treatment of patients with sepsis.

SUMMARY

Further research is required to prove that IV vitamin C and thiamine have value in the treatment of sepsis and septic shock. Although tentative preliminary evidence suggest that vitamin C may be safely administered in septic patients, further evidence is required before it can be reasonably used as an adjuvant treatment in sepsis. Thiamine is currently a more common adjuvant to treat sepsis but more clinicians should be aware of the significance of the lack of thiamine administration. Clinical judgment is required when deciding whether to apply the results of this trial at the bedside or whether to await the results of further research.

REFERENCES

1. Martin GS, Mannino DM, Eaton S, et al. The epidemiology of sepsis in the United States from 1979 through 2000. N Engl J Med 2003;348:1546.
2. Hall MJ, Williams SN, DeFrances CJ, et al. Inpatient care for septicemia or sepsis: a challenge for patients and hospitals. NCHS Data Brief 2011;62:1–8.
3. Elixhauser A, Friedman B, Stranges E. Septicemia in U.S. Hospitals, 2009. Agency for healthcare research and quality, Rockville, MD. Available at: http://www.hcup-us.ahrq.gov/reports/statbriefs/sb122.pdf. Accessed December 27, 2017.
4. Walkey AJ, Wiener RS, Lindenauer PK. Utilization patterns and outcomes associated with central venous catheter in septic shock: a population-based study. Crit Care Med 2013;41:1450.
5. Available at: https://www.cdc.gov/sepsis/datareports/index.html. Accessed December 21, 2017.
6. Fleischmann C, Scherag A, Adhikari NK, et al. Assessment of global incidence and mortality of hospital-treated sepsis. Current estimates and limitations. Am J Respir Crit Care Med 2016;193:259.
7. Angus DC, Kelley MA, Schmitz RJ, et al. Caring for the critically ill patient. Current and projected workforce requirements for care of the critically ill and patients with pulmonary disease: can we meet the requirements of an aging population? JAMA 2000;284:2762.

8. Fleischmann C, Thomas–Rueddel DO, Hartmann M, et al. Hospital incidence and mortality rates of sepsis: an analysis of hospital episode (DRG) statistics in Germany from 2007 to 2013. Dtsch Arztebl Int 2016;113(10):159–66.

9. Dugani S, Veillard J, Kissoon N. Reducing the global burden of sepsis. Can Med Assoc J 2017;189(1):E2–3.

10. Singer M, Deutschman CS, Seymour CW, et al. The third international consensus definitions for sepsis and septic shock (Sepsis-3). JAMA 2016;315(8):757–9. Available at: http://jama.jamanetwork.com/article.aspx?articleid=2492881.

11. Borrelli E, Roux-Lombard P, Grau GE, et al. Plasma concentrations of cytokines, their soluble receptors, and antioxidant vitamins can predict the development of multiple organ failure in patients at risk. Crit Care Med 1996;24:392–7.

12. Rivers E, Nguyen B, Havstad S, et al. Early goal-directed therapy in the treatment of severe sepsis and septic shock. N Engl J Med 2001;345(19):1368–77.

13. ProCESS Investigators, Yealy DM, Kellum JA, Juang DT, et al. A randomized trial of protocol based care for early septic shock. N Engl J Med 2014;370(18): 1683–93.

14. The ARISE Investigators, ANZICS Clinical Trials Group, Peake SL, Delaney A, Bailey M, et al. Goal-directed resuscitation for patients with early septic shock. N Engl J Med 2014;371(16):1496–506.

15. Mouncey PR, Osborn TM, Power GS, et al. Trial of early, goal-directed resuscitation for septic shock. N Engl J Med 2015;372(14):1301–11.

16. Castellanos-Ortega A, Suberviola B, García-Astudillo LA, et al. Impact of the surviving sepsis campaign protocols on hospital length of stay and mortality in septic shock patients: results of a three-year follow-up quasi-experimental study. Crit Care Med 2010;38:1036–43.

17. Sakr Y, Dubois MJ, De Backer D, et al. Persistent microcirculatory alterations are associated with organ failure and death in patients with septic shock. Crit Care Med 2004;32:1825–31.

18. Vincent JL, Nelson DR, Williams MD. Is worsening multiple organ failure the cause of death in patients with severe sepsis? Crit Care Med 2011;39:1050–5.

19. Wilson JX. Evaluation of vitamin C for adjuvant sepsis therapy. Antioxid Redox Signal 2013;19:2129–40.

20. FDA. FDA drug safety communication: voluntary market withdrawal of Xigris [dtrotrecogin alfa (activated)] due to failure to show a survival benefit. Available at: www.fda.gov/Drugs/DrugSafety/ucm277114.htm. Accessed December 21, 2017.

21. Marik PE, Khangoora V, Rivera R, et al. Hydrocortisone, vitamin C, and thiamine or the treatment of severe sepsis and septic shock: a retrospective before-after study. Chest 2017;151(6):1229–38.

22. Lykkesfeldt J, Poulsen HE. Is vitamin C supplementation beneficial? Lessons learned from randomised controlled trials. Br J Nutr 2010;103:1251–9.

23. Oudemans-van Straaten HM, Spoelstra-de Man AM, de Waard MC. Vitamin C revisited. Crit Care 2014;18:460.

24. Mallat J, Lemyze M, Thevenin D. Do not forget to give thiamine to your septic shock patient! J Thorac Dis 2016;8(6):1062–6.

25. Donnino MW, Carney E, Cocchi MN, et al. Thiamine deficiency in critically ill patients with sepsis. J Crit Care 2010;25:576–81.

26. Donnino MW, Andersen LW, Chase M, et al. Randomized, double-blind, placebo-controlled trial of thiamine as a metabolic resuscitator in septic shock: a pilot study. Crit Care Med 2016;44:360–7.

27. Fowler A, Syed A, Knowlson S, et al. Phase I safety trial of intravenous ascorbic acid in patients with severe sepsis. J Transl Med 2014;12:32.
28. Natarajan R, Fisher BJ, Syed A, et al. Impact of intravenous ascorbic acid infusion on novel biomarkers in patients with severe sepsis. J Pulm Respir Med 2014;4:214.
29. Zabet MH, Mohammadi M, Ramezani M, et al. Effect of high-dose ascorbic acid on vasopressor's requirement in septic shock. J Res Pharm Pract 2016;5:94–100.
30. Tanaka H, Matsuda T, Miyagantani Y, et al. Reduction of resuscitation fluid volumes in severely burned patients using ascorbic acid administration: a randomized, prospective study. Arch Surg 2000;135:326–31.

Hit or Miss? A Review of Early-Onset Sepsis in the Neonate

Monica Scheel, MSN, RN, Shannon Perkins, MSN, APRN, NNP-BC*

KEYWORDS

- Early-onset sepsis • EOS • Neonatal sepsis • Group B streptococcus • GBS
- Neonatal infection

KEY POINTS

- Neonatal sepsis carries a high morbidity and mortality rate due to the neonate's immature immune response to pathogens.
- Early-onset sepsis occurs within the first week of life.
- Identification of at-risk infants is often overlooked because clinical presentation can be subtle and vague.
- Lack of universal implementation of screening protocols leads to inconsistencies in identification and treatment of at-risk neonates.
- The role of the bedside nurse is critical in the recognition and treatment of at-risk neonates and their families.

INTRODUCTION

Infections during the neonatal period have a high incidence of developing into sepsis, which carries a high morbidity and mortality rate for this vulnerable population.[1] A major concern for health care providers is the difficulty of early diagnosis of neonatal sepsis due to inconsistent use of nationally established guidelines. Impediments to accurate diagnosis, recommended treatments, nursing management, and recommendations for addressing this high-risk condition are discussed. The primary focus is addressing early-onset sepsis (EOS) as opposed to late-onset sepsis (LOS).

DEFINITION

Neonatal sepsis can be defined as a potentially life-threatening infection occurring within the first 28 days of life. Infections may be either bacterial or viral in nature.[1]

Disclosure: The authors have nothing to disclose.
Delgado Community College-Charity School of Nursing, 450 South Claiborne Avenue, New Orleans, LA 70112, USA
* Corresponding author.
E-mail address: sperki@dcc.edu

Neonatal sepsis is separated into 2 categories: EOS and LOS. EOS occurs within the first week of life, most often within the first 3 days after birth.[2] LOS occurs after the first week of life, often from days 7 through 28 but can occur up to 90 days after birth.[1]

The primary route of transmission for EOS is vertical from the mother to the fetus during the intrapartum period, whereas LOS may be acquired through exposure to environmental contaminants from either the hospital or the community.[1] Infections in the neonate predispose the infant to sepsis development due to a weak immune system that is poorly responsive to bacteria.[3] Common infections leading to the development of sepsis include pneumonia, urosepsis, and meningitis. It is important for health care providers to suspect a diagnosis of sepsis in any neonate presenting with a fever. These infants should receive an immediate workup for sepsis and meningitis because of the rapid deterioration of the infant's physical condition.[3]

RISK FACTORS

Maternal diagnoses of intrapartum fever and chorioamnionitis are the most common factors used to identify EOS risk.[4] Chorioamnionitis is caused by vertical transmission of bacterial colonization of the uterus leading to inflammation of fetal membranes. Maternal fever and foul-smelling or cloudy amniotic fluid are the most prevalent symptoms of chorioamnionitis. The Centers for Disease Control and Prevention (CDC) guidelines allow maternal fever to be used as a surrogate for chorioamnionitis and recommend the use of neonatal antibiotics.[4] **Table 1** lists the most common risk factors requiring an EOS evaluation of the neonate.

The infant is protected within the sterile environment of the amniotic sac during pregnancy. However, pathogenic exposure from the birth canal and the environment may occur during labor and the delivery process. Neonatal immunity is received passively through transfer of maternal antibodies across the placenta, with most placental transfer occurring after 30 weeks gestation.[1] The primary form of passive immunity before birth is the transmission of immunoglobulin (Ig)G antibodies. These antibodies help protect the neonate from viruses and bacterial infections. Newborns lack IgA, IgE, and IgM antibodies because they do not readily cross the placenta. This leaves the neonate vulnerable to gram-negative organisms and certain viruses.[3] Active immunity is not developed at birth, leaving neonates susceptible to infection.

Premature infants, especially those less than 30 weeks gestation, are at higher risk of developing EOS than term infants owing to an immature immune system and lack of

Table 1	
Risk factors necessitating early-onset sepsis evaluations in the neonate	
Maternal Factors	**Fetal Factors**
Intrapartum maternal fever 38.0° – 38.2° C	Fetal tachycardia
Obstetric diagnosis of chorioamnionitis	Gestational age <37 wk
Prolonged ROM ≥24 h	Low birthweight infants
Premature rupture of membranes	Low Apgar score (<6 at 1 or 5 minutes)
GBS-positive or unknown status	Birth asphyxia
Inadequate GBS intrapartum antibiotic prophylaxis (IAP)	Meconium staining
IAP given <4 h before delivery	Congenital anomalies
No IAP given	
Poor prenatal care	

Abbreviation: ROM, rupture of membranes.
  Data from Refs.[1,5,6]

passive immunity.[1] Premature infants often have low birthweights and require invasive medical interventions, predisposing them to greater risk of infection exposure. EOS remains a primary cause of illness and death among neonates of all birthweights and gestational ages, with particularly devastating effects on premature infants.[5]

INCIDENCE

Group B streptococcus (GBS) was found to be the leading cause of EOS in the United States as early as the 1960s.[5] *Escherichia coli* is the second leading cause of neonatal EOS.[2] A maternal diagnosis of chorioamnionitis or maternal fever greater than 38°C remains the primary indicator for intrapartum antibiotic administration.[6] The CDC reported 90% of early-onset GBS sepsis manifests within the first 24 hours of life, with pneumonia, meningitis, and septicemia being the most common infections present.[7]

The incidence of GBS-related EOS is less than 1 case per 1000 live births in term infants.[3] There is a higher incidence of EOS in preterm infants of approximately 3.7 cases per 1000 live births (if <37 weeks gestation).[3] The rate for low birthweight infants (<1500 g) is approximately 11 cases per 1000 live births.[3] Despite these relatively low numbers of cases, EOS infections remain a major cause of mortality and morbidity for the neonatal population and may have long-term impacts on those who survive. **Table 2** notes highest incidence rates of EOS.

SYMPTOMS

EOS in the neonate often presents with vague, nonspecific symptoms that are easily missed.[1] Currently, there is no single set of criteria for diagnosing neonatal EOS. It is imperative that health care providers recognize risk factors and early signs of neonatal sepsis, and provide essential treatment to prevent rapid deterioration. Symptoms of EOS differ between the term infant and the premature infant.[3] Obtaining a thorough maternal history will help indicate increased risk factors requiring close assessment of the neonate for infection and sepsis development. The initial physical examination of the infant should include baseline vital signs, level of activity and alertness, muscle tone, and cardiopulmonary stability. Use of a pediatric or neonatal early warning scale scoring tool may assist with identification of high-risk infants.[1] Common signs and symptoms of neonatal EOS are listed in **Box 1**.

If meningitis is suspected, the neonate may show signs of increased irritability, jitteriness, seizures, hypertonia, and abnormal eye movements. Nuchal rigidity is often not present in the neonate and they are unable to demonstrate photophobia, although the

Table 2	
Highest incidence rates for early-onset sepsis	
Maternal	**Fetal**
Maternal chorioamnionitis or intrapartum fever >38.0°C	Premature infants <34 wk gestation
	Very low birthweight infants <2500 g
Positive GBS antenatal screening at 35–37 wk gestation	African American race
	Highest morality rate = preterm,
Prolonged rupture of membranes before delivery (>18 h)	very low birthweight
Advanced maternal age	
Caesarian delivery	

Data from Schrag S, Farley MM, Petit S, et al. Epidemiology of invasive early-onset neonatal sepsis, 2005 to 2014. Pediatrics 2016;138(6):[pii:e20162013]; and Stoll BJ. Early-onset neonatal sepsis: a continuing problem in need of novel prevention strategies. Pediatrics 2016;138(6):[pii:e20163038].

Box 1
Common signs and symptoms of neonatal early-onset sepsis

Incessant crying, unable to console

Poor feeding

Dyspnea, tachypnea, or apnea

Bradycardia or tachycardia

Hypotonia

Hypothermia less than 36°C (preterm infants)

Hyperthermia greater than 38°C (term infants)

Mottled skin color

Glucose instability

Hypoxia

Decreased responsiveness

Bulging fontanelle (suspect meningitis)

Data from Barnden J, Diamond V, Heaton PA. Recognition and management of sepsis in early infancy. Nurs Child Young People 2016;28(10):36–44.

---

infant may turn their head away from lights.[3] If the infant experiences a prolonged septic period, bleeding and clotting times will be abnormal, which may predispose the neonate to further complications. The absence of fever is not a reliable indicator of sepsis because premature neonates may not have the capability to generate a febrile response to infectious processes.[1] These nonspecific symptoms of EOS are often missed opportunities in accurately diagnosing and treating neonatal sepsis.

DIAGNOSIS

A focused history and astute clinical evaluation are the basis for diagnosing neonatal EOS. Ascertaining risk factors from the maternal history and clinical symptoms of the infant enable the health care provider to perform a thorough EOS assessment and workup. Components of a focused history are included in **Box 2**.

Box 2
Components of a focused history

Maternal health history

GBS screening results

Intrapartum antibiotic prophylaxis given to mother during labor

Duration of membrane rupture

Infections in prior pregnancies

Birth history

Feeding tolerance of newborn

Onset of respiratory distress in the newborn after than 4 hours of life

Data from Barnden J, Diamond V, Heaton PA. Recognition and management of sepsis in early infancy. Nurs Child Young People 2016;28(10):36–44.

It must be reemphasized that infection in a neonate can be present without obvious clinical symptoms; therefore, infants in high-risk categories should receive a detailed sepsis workup. **Table 3** lists common diagnostic tests included in a neonatal EOS evaluation.

One of the main difficulties in identifying newborns at risk for EOS is the occurrence of bacteremia among infants born to mothers who screen GBS negative.[8] Rescreening GBS negative mothers with real-time nucleic-acid amplification testing at the time of presentation for delivery could remediate this problem; however, this is not deemed to be a cost-efficient practice.[8] The development and implementation of a GBS vaccine may provide the safest and most efficient approach to the neonatal GBS EOS problem.[8] Substantial variation remains in newborn EOS risk assessment, which affects the definition of risk, the level of medical intervention required, and the impact on mother–infant separation.[4] Identifying and implementing an optimal approach to EOS risk assessment could positively affect the care of a large proportion of newborns.

The CDC established national guidelines for prevention of neonatal GBS disease in 1996 and revised these guidelines in 2002 and 2010. The guidelines contain recommendations for evaluation, treatment, and management of GBS in the mother and the infant. In 2010, collaborative efforts between the CDC, the American Academy of Pediatrics (AAP), the Committee on Fetus and Newborn, the American College of Nurse-Midwives, the American College of Obstetricians and Gynecologists, and the Committee on Infectious Diseases set forth to revise and endorse a single set of national guidelines for detecting and managing early-onset GBS disease in neonates.[9] The approved algorithm is available for review at https://www.cdc.gov/groupbstrep/guidelines/downloads/secondary-prevention.pdf.

Despite these national guidelines, wide variation still exists in clinical practice regarding approaches to sepsis screening and management in the neonate.[8]

Table 3
Diagnostic testing for early-onset sepsis

Blood Cultures	Minimum of 1 mL Sample Required[3]
Complete blood count	Including white blood cell differential and platelet count at birth and/or a 6–12 h of life[6]
Chest radiograph	Indicated with respiratory abnormalities or when source of infection remains unidentified[6]
Lumbar puncture	May be deferred in critically ill infants until their physical condition stabilizes[6] Focus specifically on the white blood cell count and differential[3]
Urinalysis and urine culture	Urine culture important even when urinalysis is normal because newborns do not store urine in the bladder long enough to produce nitrates in response to bacteria[3]
C-reactive protein	Indicates inflammation, often used as an indicator of when to discontinue antibiotics, instead of when to start them[3]
Skin and vesicle swabs	If herpes or varicella suspected, puncture vesicle and take swab by scraping bottom of the lesion[3]

Data from Rubarth LB, Christensen CM, Riley C. Bacterial sepsis in the neonate. Nurse Pract 2017;42(9):25–32; and Center for Disease Control and Prevention (CDC). Questions and answers about implementing the 2010 guidelines for neonatal providers: algorithm for secondary prevention of early-onset group-B streptococcal (GBS) disease among newborns. CDC.Gov 2016. Available at: https://www.cdc.gov/groupbstrep/clinicians/qas-neonatal.html. Accessed January 4, 2018.

Confusion regarding initial interpretation of recommendations among the CDC and the AAP guidelines was noted as a primary source of variation in guideline usage.[4] This variation in evaluation, diagnosis, and management of GBS EOS in the neonate under-scores the importance of stricter adherence to a single set of national guidelines to improve rates of accurate diagnosis and early treatment of EOS.

Neonatal providers expressed the following concerns as a basis for nonadherence to established guidelines: (1) low risk (0.4 cases per 1000 births) of GBS infection to infants of GBS-positive mothers in the absence of additional risk factors, including fever or prolonged rupture of membranes[8]; (2) development of resistance to first-line beta-lactam therapies used as prophylactic treatment of GBS[2]; and (3) neonatal exposure to intrapartum antibiotics may increase risk of sepsis from non-GBS patho-gens, especially *E coli*.[2] However, adherence to the 2010 CDC guidelines on preven-tion may eliminate the need for up to 25% of current EOS screening, improve methods for distinguishing high-risk infants, decrease mortality and morbidity rates, decrease incidence of early-onset GBS sepsis, and improve outcomes for neonates.[5] Inclusion of the GBS EOS protocol established by the CDC and AAP, as a core measure to be monitored by the Joint Commission, may provide the impetus for health care agencies to adhere to a standardized approach for neonatal EOS identification, treatment, and management. The main identification of infants with possible EOS is based on obstet-ric and neonatal risk factors and the condition of the infant at birth. Evaluating the infant's condition remains challenging and depends on clinical expertise.[5]

TREATMENT

As stated previously, there remains substantial variation in risk identification, evaluation, and treatment of neonatal EOS.[4] Reported management does either more or less than national standards recommend. Although it is important to tailor practice to account for local resources and structures of care, variations in decisions to start and stop antibi-otics among newborns under the same clinical circumstances represent unnecessary deviations in management that could have a negative impact on the newborn.[4]

The primary goal of antibiotic therapy is to adequately cover the most likely patho-gens while preventing antibiotic overuse and resistance.[3] The site of microbial entry is not always easy to identify in neonatal sepsis; therefore, initiating antibiotic therapy with broad-spectrum coverage is desired until therapy can be narrowed because of culture and sensitivity testing, usually after 36 to 48 hours of treatment.[6] Duration of antimicrobial therapy ranges between 7 and 21 days. Dosages and intervals vary by gestational age, postnatal age, weight, and depend on the suspected site-specific location of the infection.[3]

Antibiotics have various mechanisms of action and are frequently used in combina-tion for better efficacy, or for the treatment and prevention of microbial resistance.[3] This is often referred to as double-coverage. The primary purpose is to attack the pathogen by killing it before the organism's ability to develop resistance. Certain an-tibiotics should be avoided in the neonatal population owing to the increased risk of adverse reactions, including (1) trimethoprim-sulfamethoxazole (Bactrim), (2) ceftriax-one, and (3) tetracycline.[3]

Most infants exposed to intrapartum antibiotics were given beta-lactams (eg. ampi-cillin or penicillin) or cephalosporins.[6,10] Many antimicrobials are not approved by the US Food and Drug Administration for use in infants, yet primary research and literature supports the safety and efficacy for use of these medications. Health care providers are encouraged to review dosing recommendations frequently because research is always ongoing with newer antibiotics.[3]

Concern about risks of prolonged early neonatal antibiotic exposure has been recognized as among the reasons for variation in sepsis management by health care providers.[2] Risks of early neonatal antibiotic exposure can lead to increases in (1) LOS, (2) necrotizing enterocolitis, (3) fungal infections, (4) recurrent wheezing disorders, (5) permanent and severe hearing loss associated with aminoglycosides (eg, gentamicin), (6) impact on the development of the intestinal microbiome (normal distribution and function of cellular structures within the body) with resulting risk of gastrointestinal disease, and (7) death.[2]

Selection of the appropriate antimicrobial therapy requires careful consideration of various factors.[10] If sepsis is strongly suspected, the National Institute for Health and Care Excellence has developed guidelines for treatment initiation, which includes[1]

- Starting treatment with intravenous (IV) antibiotics before receiving the results of diagnostic tests
- Administering antibiotics within 1 hour of therapy initiation
- Reviewing the antibiotic course length at 36 hours (health care providers may consider discontinuing IV antibiotics if the infant remains well and blood culture remains negative).

Treatment modalities in EOS may include but are not restricted to the following[1,4]:

- Antibiotics, antivirals, and immunoglobulins
- Isolation (especially when MRSA and other specific infections are present)
- Antipyretics (the drug of choice is acetaminophen, prescribed based on body weight)
- Fluids and supportive management (focused on maintaining stable blood glucose and electrolyte levels through fluid resuscitation, IV parenteral nutrition, or nasogastric tube feedings)
- Cardiopulmonary support (focused on stabilizing blood pressure with inotropes to maintain urine output, as well as administer oxygen and ventilatory assistance as needed)
- Maintaining neutral body temperature (may require placement in an incubator or overhead warmer to avoid shivering or overheating)
- Close monitoring (may require transfer to neonatal intensive care unit).

Antivirals and immunoglobulins may be indicated for severe viral sepsis with herpes simplex virus (HSV) or varicella.[1] Infants with HSV infection should be treated with IV acyclovir (60 mg/kg/d). If varicella is present, the infant will require IV varicella zoster immunoglobulin to prevent the serious complication of varicella pneumonia.[1]

NURSING MANAGEMENT

It is important to consider the possibility of EOS in the differential diagnosis of ill or at-risk newborns because symptoms of EOS are often vague and nonspecific. Early identification leads to appropriate treatment, enabling better outcomes for the neonate. Nurses play a vital role in managing infants with EOS through early detection, initiating treatment, ongoing monitoring, and supporting families.

Nursing management for EOS involves regular observations, use of a neonatal early warning scale, monitoring fluid balance, supporting maternal-infant bonding, and breastfeeding. Some degree of mother–infant separation is required for EOS evaluation, and separation for the entire duration of antibiotic therapy is required at times.[8]

The nurse assumes a leading role in ensuring that bonding between mother and infant is firmly established, as well as expertly addressing the psychological needs of the parents. Psychological support for the parents should address 3 main aspects:

- Explanation: Parents need an understanding of why infections arise because they often feel guilty about having done something wrong, resulting in the neonate's illness.[1]
- Communication: Establishing regular contact with the family allows nurses to keep parents informed and involved in their newborn's care. When parents are directly involved in the practical aspects of care (eg, diaper changes, feedings) they are likely better to cope with the emotional trauma of having a sick child.[9]
- Trust: Consistent communication assists in the building of trust between nurses and parents, which is an essential part of providing family-centered care.[1]

Parents often experience depression, anxiety, stress, and loss of control.[1] They vacillate between feelings of inclusion and exclusion related to the provision of health care for their infant. Nursing interventions that promote positive psychosocial outcomes are needed to decrease these parental feelings. Interventions should be focused on delivering family-centered, developmentally supportive care. The role of the nurse in meeting the emotional needs of the parents is of paramount importance.[1] **Box 3** highlights implications for nursing practice.

PROGNOSIS

When an infection is detected early and treated effectively, the long-term prognosis for infants is improved.[1] Infants who develop severe cases of EOS may require long-term outpatient follow-up to assess for developmental delays, achievement of proper developmental milestones, and persistent neurologic problems. If meningitis or encephalitis develops with EOS, particularly when associated with HSV, GBS, or *E coli*, there may be long-term neurologic complications from the infection.[1] Although

---

Box 3
Implications for nursing practice for neonatal sepsis

- Remain aware of the various signs and symptoms of sepsis in early infancy.
- Ensure regular monitoring and a prompt medical review of a newborn whose clinical condition deteriorates.
- When sepsis is suspected, antibiotic therapy should be administered in 1 hour.
- Ensure blood and cerebrospinal fluid cultures are checked in a timely manner and that antibiotics are discontinued when indicated.
- Arrange for timely transfer to a specialized unit (neonatal intensive care unit) when necessary.
- Ensure parents are involved in the care of their infant as much as possible.
- Encourage parents to immunize their infants, even if they have suffered a serious infection in the newborn period.
- Educate parents about fever and promote safe use of a single antipyretic agent.
- Collaborate with medical professional colleagues regarding any concerns about suspected developmental delay, even when this is an incidental finding.

Data from Barnden J, Diamond V, Heaton PA. Recognition and management of sepsis in early infancy. Nurs Child Young People 2016;28(10):36–44.

mortality is highest among very low birthweight infants infected with *E coli*, birthweight, pathogens, and mortality are interconnected. Approximately 6% of EOS survivors are reported to have long-term sequelae at time of hospital discharge.[5] If a developmental delay is suspected, the child should be referred to the appropriate pediatric specialist service. As previously mentioned, an increasing number of studies associate exposure to antibiotics early in life with a negative impact on subsequent child health. One of the most significant findings is the condition known as dysbiosis, which is an unhealthy change in the normal bacterial ecology of the body mediated by antibiotic exposures.[2] The potential long-term consequences of this can markedly affect an infant's future health status. However, notably, EOS remains among the leading causes of infant death in the United States.[2]

RECOMMENDATIONS

Further study of pathogens causing EOS is warranted due to the potential negative impact of complications on the infant's neurodevelopment and issues affecting normal microbial activity. The development of an effective maternal immunization against invasive pathogens could prevent disease in the mother, fetus, and the newborn. A specific vaccine for GBS may prevent both EOS and LSO and mitigate other adverse outcomes of pregnancy, including stillbirth, prematurity, and culture-negative sepsis.[5]

Utilization of the CDC guidelines for the use of intrapartum antibiotic prophylaxis to prevent perinatal GBS infection has led to a significant decrease in the incidence of both overall and GBS-specific neonatal EOS.[8] Nationwide adherence to the CDC guidelines as the best standards of care for management of EOS should be implemented.

Establishing neonatal EOS as a quality indicator for the Joint Commission can serve a twofold purpose. First and foremost, it will serve as a driving force for health care providers and agencies to incorporate the guidelines as set forth by the CDC and AAP. This will serve to decrease the wide variation among practitioners in the evaluation, diagnosis, and medical management required for septic newborns. Adherence to a set algorithm will enable consistency in the approach of caring for this vulnerable population. Second, attaching a financial incentive for adherence to the guidelines, by way of a national quality scoring on meeting the quality indicators (similar to those currently in place for conditions such as heart failure and pneumonia) will ensure a sustained impetus toward consistency in caring for EOS patients. Quality scores must be published on specific hospital Web sites to allow public viewing of how well the organization is meeting this indicator for quality patient care. This will drive hospitals to assume a pay-for-performance role in providing the highest quality of care for this patient population.

SUMMARY

Great strides have been made in the identification and treatment of neonatal EOS; however, the fight is far from over. Universal adherence to CDC guidelines for GBS EOS sepsis by health care professionals is paramount to the rapid identification and management of this vulnerable population.[8] Bedside nurses are an integral part of the health care team because they are often the first to encounter subtle clinical changes in the neonate. Early identification and treatment is essential, especially for premature and very low birthweight infants, because they have the highest morbidity and mortality rates from EOS.[5] Through continued education, vigilance, and family-centered focus, health care providers can prevent missed opportunities in addressing neonatal EOS.

REFERENCES

1. Barnden J, Diamond V, Heaton PA. Recognition and management of sepsis in early infancy. Nurs Child Young People 2016;28(10):36–44.
2. Schrag S, Farley M, Petit S, et al. Epidemiology of invasive early-onset neonatal sepsis, 2005 to 2014. Pediatrics 2016;138(6) [pii:e20162013].
3. Rubarth LB, Christensen CM, Riley C. Bacterial sepsis in the neonate. Nurse Pract 2017;42(9):25–32.
4. Mukhopadhyay S, Taylor JA, Von Kohorn I, et al. Variation in sepsis evaluation across a national network of nurseries. Pediatrics 2017;139(3) [pii:e20162845].
5. Stoll BJ. Early-onset neonatal sepsis: a continuing problem in need of novel prevention strategies. Pediatrics 2016;138(6) [pii:e20163038].
6. Questions and answers about implementing the 2010 guidelines for neonatal providers: algorithm for secondary prevention of early-onset group-B streptococcal (GBS) disease among newborns. 2016. Available at: cdc.gov/groupbstrep/clinicians/qas-neonatal.html.
7. Algorithm for secondary prevention of early-onset group B streptococcal (GBS) disease among newborns. 2010. Available at: https://www.cdc.gov/groupbstrep/guidelines/downloads/secondary-prevention.pdf.
8. Mukhopadhyay S, Eichenwald EC, Puopolo KM. Neonatal early-onset sepsis evaluations among well-appearing infants: projected impact of changes in CDC GBS guidelines. J Perinatol 2013;33:198–205.
9. Brady MT, Polin RA. Prevention and management of infants with suspected or proven neonatal sepsis. Pediatrics 2013;132(1):166–8. Available at: http://pediatrics.aappublications.org/content/132/1/166.
10. Committee on Infectious Diseases, Committee on Fetus and Newborn, Baker CJ, Byington CL, Polin RA. Policy statement—Recommendations for the prevention of perinatal Group B Streptococcal (GBS) disease. Pediatrics 2011;128(3):611–6.

Simulation to Manage the Septic Patient in the Intensive Care Unit

Alison H. Davis, PhD, RN, CHSE[a],*, Sherri P. Hayes, MSN, RN, CCRN[b]

KEYWORDS

- Sepsis • Severe sepsis • Septic shock • High-fidelity human patient simulation
- Simulation

KEY POINTS

- Sepsis and septic shock are complex clinical conditions with high rates of morbidity and mortality.
- Nurses are directly involved with patient care and must have knowledge of evidence-based guidelines for the sepsis patient.
- High-fidelity human patient simulation (HF-HPSim) is used to increase the quality and quantity of student learning experiences in nursing education, while providing an experiential and safe learning environment.
- With its complexity and associated risks to patients, sepsis and septic shock are appropriate content to be taught with HF-HPSim.

Health care reform and advancing technologies in clinical practice and education are influencing today's health care professional student (eg, nurse, physician, respiratory therapist) to acquire clinical skills before graduation to care for patients in diverse health care settings. Today's health care settings have increasing complexity regarding technology and level of patient acuity. All health care graduates, especially nurses, who are directly involved with patient care must transition into practice as practitioners who can provide safe, quality, timely, and competent care.

Sepsis and septic shock are associated with high morbidity and mortality rates. Most patients with a diagnosis of sepsis are cared for by the health care team in the intensive care unit. However, evidence-based recommendations now indicate the need for screening of patients in the emergency departments and general medical floors.[1–3] Nurses provide direct patient care in these areas. Therefore, nurses can

Disclosure Statement: The authors have nothing to disclose.
[a] Louisiana State University Health Sciences Center, School of Nursing, 1900 Gravier Street, Office 506, New Orleans, LA 70112, USA; [b] Louisiana State University Health Sciences Center, School of Nursing, 1900 Gravier Street, Office 504, New Orleans, LA 70112, USA
* Corresponding author.
E-mail address: adav27@lsuhsc.edu

https://doi.org/10.1016/j.cnc.2018.05.005
0899-5885/18/© 2018 Elsevier Inc. All rights reserved.
ccnursing.theclinics.com

be a patient's first line of defense against sepsis through early recognition, comprehensive nursing assessments, and knowledge of evidence-based treatment plans for sepsis. To facilitate positive patient outcomes regarding sepsis, simulation, specifically, high-fidelity human patient simulation (HF-HPSim), can be used as an educational tool in nursing education. HF-HPSim is a student-centered, experiential, educational pedagogy that engages and prepares learners for real-world practice without risk of harm.[4]

SEPSIS
Definitions of Sepsis

Sepsis is defined as "a life-threatening organ dysfunction resulting from a dysregulated host response to infection."[3] A subset of sepsis associated with circulatory, cellular, and metabolic alterations is considered septic shock, with the inclusion of higher mortality rates than sepsis alone.[3]

Overview

A source of infection (abscess, infected necrosis, infected intravascular access devices, oral decontamination with ventilated patients leading to ventilator-associated pneumonia) stimulates the innate immune system, activates white blood cells with an endothelial response, and releases mediators or cytokines in the process of sepsis.[1] The activation of this process results in a multitude of physiologic changes, including vasodilation, increased expression of adhesion molecules, capillary permeability, clot formation, and decreased fibrinolysis.[1] The overactivity of mediators contributes to endothelial cell damage, microcapillary permeability changes, capillary leak, vasodilation, and hypotension.[1] The progression of sepsis when not recognized or treated early leads to sepsis, septic shock, and the development of multiple organ system dysfunction.

To assist health care clinicians in managing sepsis through early recognition and treatment, and to improve patient outcomes and decrease mortality rates, new evidence-based guidelines have been released. The Surviving Sepsis Campaign implemented in 2012, with updates in 2016, organizes recommendations for sepsis care into 3 categories: (1) recommendations targeting the management of severe sepsis, (2) recommendations targeting high-priority general care, and (3) pediatric considerations.[1–3] These guidelines identify aims of early recognition, early treatment, and reduction of morbidity and mortality rates surrounding sepsis and its progression.

Nurses are a crucial component of the health care team. Nurses can integrate the new evidence-based recommendations surrounding sepsis into practice, thus improving the care of patients who are at risk for developing sepsis.

SIMULATION
Definitions of Simulation

Simulation is defined as "a student or group of students providing care for a patient who is represented by a mannequin, an actor, or a standardized patient, depending on the clinical situation."[5] The clinical situation can be represented through a scripted, predetermined scenario or an unscripted on-the-fly scenario. The clinical scenario is followed by a debriefing session. The debriefing session is an opportunity for learners and educators to reflect on the scenario as it unfolded. Constructive feedback is provided by educators and is used as a complement and experiential application to didactic and clinical learning.

Simulation is further described by the level of fidelity or realism represented by the mannequin (simulator) or standardized patient used for the scenario. High-fidelity simulation is a "patient-care scenario that uses a standardized patient or a full-body patient simulator that can be programmed to respond to affective and psychomotor changes, such as breathing chest action."[6] Medium-fidelity or moderate-fidelity simulation is a "patient-care scenario that uses a full-body simulator with installed human qualities such as breath sounds without chest rise."[6] Low-fidelity simulation uses task trainers or "part of a mannequin designed for a specific psychomotor skill, for example, an IV [intravenous] arm."[6]

Overview

Since the 1990s, HF-HPSim has grown into a well-established teaching pedagogy in nursing education.[7] With a shortage of clinical sites, advances in technology, decreasing costs of simulators, and an increase in simulation research, nursing programs throughout the United States are increasingly using HF-HPSim. In nursing education, HF-HPSim is used to increase the quality and quantity of student learning experiences; especially in difficult-to-access, vulnerable patient populations and/or if safety of the student or faculty is in question.[8,9]

Simulation usage in nursing education matches the shift from an emphasis on teaching to an emphasis on learning for students.[4] Nursing faculty act as the facilitators of learning by encouraging learners to "discover, or construct, knowledge and meaning."[10] Aligned with this shift is the experiential learning cycle that is supported through the use of HF-HPSim.[11] The experiential learning cycle is

A continuous process in which knowledge is created by transforming experience. Individuals have a concrete experience (reflective observation), they derive meaning (abstract conceptualization) from the experience, and they try out or apply (active experimentation) the meaning they've created thus continuing the cycle with another concrete experience.[10]

HF-HPSim provides this experience for learners as they add new knowledge to their previous knowledge.

Benefits of High-Fidelity Human Patient Simulation

HF-HPSim provides nursing students with the ability to experience realistic, high-risk scenarios without harm to themselves or the faculty.[8] HF-HPSim provides students an opportunity to use the cognitive, psychomotor, and affective domains of learning. Research indicates that, through the use of HF-HPSim, nursing students improved in a multitude of areas, including

- Self-confidence
- Self-efficacy
- Satisfaction with learning
- Critical thinking skills
- Clinical judgment
- Clinical skills
- Clinical performance
- Safe medication administration
- Leadership skills.[5,12–21]

"Simulations can provide an innovative, experiential approach to teaching that actively involves students in their learning process. By interacting with simulations, the learner is required to use a higher order of learning than simply mimicking the teacher role model."[22] Faculty provide a supportive role to learners in the form of cues or technical support.[8] Active observation of students allows faculty to provide real-time positive feedback during debriefing, which enables learners to experience the so-called lightbulb moment as they reflect on their actions, make connections between theory and practice, gain confidence, and begin to comprehend the cause-and-effect relationship of critical thinking during the simulation.[21,23]

After nursing school, HF-HPSim has been used to assist new graduate nurses transition into practice. As baccalaureate-prepared nurses graduate, they are prepared as nurse generalists.[24] However, with the current nursing shortage, new graduates are accepting positions in specialty areas, including critical care. For new graduate nurses, employment in specialty areas immediately after graduation can affect their readiness to practice. The decrease in readiness to practice has been noted as a lack of confidence and clinical skills that lasts up to a year after graduation.[25] These factors lead to decreased job satisfaction for new graduate nurses and promote intrinsic concerns regarding the ability to ensure safe patient care. Ultimately, new graduate nurses experience low morale and end up leaving positions or the profession of nursing entirely.[25]

To address decreased readiness to practice, the literature supports nurse residency programs that include HF-HPSim. HF-HPSim provides the hands-on aspect of skill attainment in a simulation clinical environment. Because it is a practice discipline, nursing must be taught in classrooms and in clinical settings. This is true for new graduate nurses because knowledge gained in an academic setting at the generalist level can be refined or built on in the simulated setting. HF-HPSim in a residency program "can bridge the gap between knowledge already gained in academic curricula and skills needed to care for multiple, complex patients."[25] HF-HPSim is planned for the level of the student or the new graduate to ensure knowledge gain or refinement, and clinical refinement, leading to expertise through feedback in a facilitator-led debriefing.

HIGH-FIDELITY HUMAN PATIENT SIMULATION AS AN EDUCATIONAL TOOL FOR SEPSIS MANAGEMENT IN THE INTENSIVE CARE UNIT

Sepsis is a complex care issue that should be treated as a medical emergency.[26] As a safe learning environment, HF-HPSim can provide students or recent graduates with a range of clinical scenarios that are rare and/or considered high-risk, such as resuscitation and critical events (ie, sepsis). By exposing new graduate nurses to these unlikely and risky clinical scenarios in HF-HPSim, these clinical situations can be experienced directly. In HF-HPSim, "the instructor, preceptor, or staff nurse does not take over."[27] HF-HPSim allows the new graduate to develop critical thinking skills in complex clinical situations without the risk of harm to themselves or patients.[5]

Developing a High-Fidelity Human Patient Simulation

Nursing educators are only limited by their creativity when designing an HF-HPSim. Scenarios can be designed to meet the needs of varying levels and experience of learners in diverse settings by using multiple patients, complex patients, advanced clinical technologies, and intradisciplinary or interdisciplinary aspects. Prelicensure, advanced practice, orientation programs, and continuing education programs can all use HF-HPSim as a teaching pedagogy to meet learning objectives and/or outcomes. However, there are considerations when integrating HF-HPSim into health care education, including new graduate nurse education. These considerations are

- Using the science of learning correlated into simulation pedagogy
- Identifying best practices of HF-HPSim for learners and teachers
- Using and promoting a learner-centered approach versus a teacher-centered approach
- Providing a safe, nonthreatening environment (physically and psychologically) for new graduate nurses to practice within their scope and as a member of the health care team
- Providing an orientation (learners and teachers) to simulation pedagogy to optimize learning outcomes
- Including the concept of collaborative practice, partnerships, and consortiums for the promotion of a shared mental model
- Providing faculty development to ensure integration into current educational practices
- Developing or refining a comprehensive evaluation plan measuring learning objectives or outcomes and competencies of the new nurse graduate
- Developing a plan of research surrounding clinical simulation pedagogy to aid in identification and refinement of best practices of simulation while contributing to the science of nursing.[4]

Advance planning is required to use HF-HPSim successfully as a teaching pedagogy. Complementary to the considerations previously listed, planning should include the assessment of the availability of resources, curriculum needs (traditional or as part of a nurse residency program), preparation of students, and simulation development for faculty.

HF-HPSim requires physical space to accommodate learners, faculty, and equipment for the simulation activity, as well as debriefing. Equipment includes technology to support the high-fidelity simulator and equipment to mimic the clinical unit that the scenario would take place for the learner, whether this is a medical-surgical unit or an intensive care unit. An electronic health record should be available to increase fidelity. Audiovisual equipment should also be available for projection of mannequin vital signs and supporting documentation seen in the clinical setting, such as laboratory results and radiologic images. Additionally, audiovisual equipment can provide recordings of the HF-HPSim scenario to be used during debriefing for reflection and analysis of actions that occurred.

Before an HF-HPSim scenario can be conceptualized, a needs assessment and analysis should be performed to determine the learning objectives to be met. In general, 4 to 5 objectives are sufficient to guide a successful simulation.[28] In the case of new graduate nurses, an analysis of a residency program curricula or review of current research regarding readiness to practice provides faculty with direction for content areas for HF-HPSim scenarios. "Only 10% of nurse executives believed that new graduate nurses (NGNs) were fully prepared to practice safely and effectively. NGNs agreed with nurse executives that they lack confidence and adequate skills for up to a year after graduation."[25] To design an HF-HPSim scenario that covers identified objectives, the faculty must consider "who the learners are, why they learn, what they learn, and how they learn."[10] These considerations by faculty will provide a plan for meeting the identified objectives through an HF-HPSim scenario. The most important component for designing a simulation is the identification of clear learning objectives that guide and drive the scenario and debriefing.[28]

To meet the identified learning objectives, faculty should use an organized approach when planning the HF-HPSim scenario. The National League for Nursing (NLN) Jeffries Simulation Framework was developed to identify components of the HF-HPSim scenario process, and the relationship between these components and the design, implementation, and evaluation of simulation activities.[8,29] The NLN Jeffries Simulation Framework explicates the major constructs integral to simulation-based education. Specific components include the use of clear objectives, information, learner support, problem-solving, fidelity, and debriefing.[8,29]

While considering developing an HF-HPSim scenario, faculty should be aware that there are commercially available scenarios from a variety of simulation companies and/or manufacturers. However, if there is not an available HF-HPSim scenario on the selected content, faculty need to develop the scenario at the level appropriate for the learner. The HF-HPSim scenario should represent a real-life patient care situation, allowing the learner to build on and advance their understanding, confidence, and competence surrounding the simulated condition when it occurs in the clinical arena.[28] There should be a clear connection between learning objectives and the HF-HPSim scenario. Faculty can draw from prior clinical experiences and expertise when developing scenarios for accurate depictions of events and responses. If the faculty does not have clinical expertise in a content area, a content expert should be consulted.

With a newly developed HF-HPSim scenario, events and responses can be written as a script with progressing states or phases that contain nursing behaviors (cognitive, psychomotor, and possibly affective) that learners must meet to progress through the scenario. However, instead of a script, faculty may choose to follow a bulleted outline of expected nursing behavior or even a branching or nonbranching diagram representative of a clinical decision tree. The format of the scenario is not as imperative as the representation of reality that would unfold in a clinical setting as decisions are made and responses are presented to the learners in the appropriate sequence of real-time events.

Faculty should consider the skills included in the HF-HPSim scenario, as well as the predetermined objectives to establish a timeframe for the experience. There is no consensus on the correct timeframe for an HF-HPSim. Some simulation experts recommend 15 to 20-minute scenarios, whereas others prefer 7-minute scenarios. The time allocated for debriefing following the HF-HPSim should be at least as long as the scenario, if not twice as long, to allow adequate time for reflection.[28]

Newly developed HF-HPSim scenarios should be approached as an author writing a story (clinical story in this case). Every story has a beginning, middle, and conclusion or end. The process is as follows.

In the case of a simulation scenario, one should consider the beginning as everything that occurs before the students enter the room to start the simulation. The middle of the story is what occurs when the students are in the simulated experience. The ending or conclusion begins while the students are still in the simulation room and extends until the end of the debriefing session.[28]

The HF-HPSim scenario must be written to allow the learner to play an integral part in the outcome while interacting with the experience. HF-HPSim scenarios are time-limited, so the entire story must be completed or experienced by the learner. However, if a learner does not complete all learning objectives, debriefing can be used to finish the story and solidify knowledge.[28] Faculty decide when the learner should enter the HF-HPSim scenario and provide information to the learner to enhance this experience or background information. This background information (medical record or history and physical) can be provided to learners well before or immediately before the simulation. The simulated patient should be determined and be included at the beginning of the HF-HPSim scenario. The simulated patient should be described in detail, with appropriate clothing, equipment, and props (ie, moulage), so that the patient becomes realistic to the learners. The middle of the HF-HPSim is when the scenario delves into clinical reality with enough complexity of situation and uncertainty for learners to make clinical decisions and guide the outcome of the scenario.[28] The amount of uncertainty requiring clinical decision-making should match the level and abilities of the learner to work through the HF-HPSim and meet the learning objectives. Even experienced simulation faculty cannot anticipate all learner actions that might occur during an HF-HPSim. HF-HPSim has been described as inherently unpredictable and dynamic, therefore, the faculty writing the scenario and running the scenario must be content experts to "know what would happen next in real life and be able to quickly adjust the scenario to incorporate these unpredictable events."[28] The end of the HF-HPSim allows learners to process the consequences of their actions and occurs after the interaction with the simulated patient.[28] Most of the end of the HF-HPSim occurs in the debriefing room using the learning objectives to guide the debriefing.

Learner preparation for HF-HPSim is essential even if the learner has experienced HF-HPSim as a nursing student. The ground rules for HF-HPSim must be explained because the learner is now a graduated nurse versus a nursing student. Expectations should be higher and in line with the role of the nurse generalist so that the learning objectives can be met and so knowledge is built on while gaining confidence with new experiences.[24]

The role of the faculty in HF-HPSim is that of the facilitator of knowledge versus the provider of new knowledge. This is unlike the traditional classroom setting and faculty must be aware of this difference in teaching with HF-HPSim.[10] The faculty role does vary depending on the complexity of the scenario but must be maintained at a facilitator level so that the experiential learning process is successful for learners.[11] Faculty can provide learner support through cuing or prompting as needed throughout the HF-HPSim, and as the facilitator of the debriefing process.

Debriefing follows an HF-HPSim scenario and is a key design feature faculty should consider. All simulation-based learning experiences should include a planned debriefing session that promotes reflective thinking because learning depends on the integration of experience and reflection.[11,30] Reflective thinking is not an innate ability but can be taught with time and the guidance of an effective facilitator who has a thorough understanding of the HF-HPSim scenario.[30] Research has shown that debriefing to promote reflection is the cornerstone of simulation-based education and is considered the most important component of the simulated experience through the provision of experiential learning.[30,31]

In developing an HF-HPSim, several debriefing methodologies exist. These include but are not limited to the gather, analyze, summarize (GAS) model, the Debriefing Assessment for Simulation in Healthcare (DASH), and Debriefing for Meaningful Learning.[31] Even though these methodologies differ slightly, the recurrent theme is that faculty should provide learners with an opportunity to describe what the simulation experience was like for them, including a guided review of the patient and objectives, the identification and categorization of thought processes, reinforcement of teaching, and correction of misconceptions through active participation.[10]

Using a High-Fidelity Human Patient Simulation Scenario Template

When developing an HF-HPSim scenario, faculty can modify an existing scenario or begin with a blank canvas. Faculty who are experienced or new to scenario development can both benefit from the use of a standardized template. A template provides a consistent guide ensuring no key elements are overlooked during development. There are commercially available templates; however, a template can also be created as long as essential parts of the HF-HPSim are included. **Box 1** includes the essential components of an HF-HPSim.

APPLICATION OF HIGH-FIDELITY HUMAN PATIENT SIMULATION FOR SEPSIS MANAGEMENT IN THE INTENSIVE CARE UNIT

To provide an experiential learning environment where there is no risk of harm to patients, a sepsis HF-HPSim is appropriate because the "incidence, hospitalization rates, and mortality of sepsis remains one of the leading causes of morbidity and mortality worldwide."[1] As a high-risk, complex diagnosis, sepsis can be developed into a topic for an HF-HPSim.

HF-HPSim scenarios can address pediatric and adult patients with sepsis. An HS-HPSim scenario can reflect clinical guidelines for the management of sepsis and septic shock with interventions following the essential components of an HF-HPSim scenario template.

High-Fidelity Human Patient Simulation Scenario Examples

The first example involves the care of a 72-year-old man with sepsis and a history of Alzheimer disease. Mr Smith has been a resident in an area nursing home for the past 10 years because his family is unable to care for him. He has a medical history of mild hypertension with blood pressures running 140 to 160 over 85 to 95. His normal mental status is that he responds to his name and follows commands appropriately. Mr Smith

---

Box 1
Essential components of a high-fidelity human patient simulation

1. HF-HPSim scenario title

2. Learning objectives

3. Equipment and supplies, including simulator preparation information (eg, moulage, simulator programming, documentation or electronic health record)

4. Level of complexity

5. Target learner group

6. Simulated patient name, age, gender, weight

7. Overview or synopsis

8. Patient history

9. Report for learners

10. Health care provider orders

11. Learning performance measures (ie, clinical decisions, nursing skills, and identified learner responses)

12. Estimated scenario time

13. Estimated debriefing time

14. References

Data from Aschenbrenner DS, Milgrom LB, Settles J. Designing simulation scenarios to promote learning. In Jeffries PR, editor. Simulation in nursing education: from conceptualization to evaluation. New York: National League for Nursing; 2012. p. 43–76; and CAE Healthcare. SCE development form. 2012. Available at: https://caehealthcare.com/media/files/Academy-Documentation/SCE-Development-Form.pdf. Accessed January 4, 2018.

Table 1
Abridged adult sepsis, septic shock high-fidelity human patient simulation scenario

State Description	Events or Simulator Actions	Health Care Provider Orders	Learner Expected Behaviors	Faculty Activities
1. ED Assessment (baseline)	HR = 122 BP = 88/62 RR = 26, slightly labored SpO2 = 91% on room air Breath sounds = clear Urine output = 10 mL/h dark, brown, cloudy	1. Admit to ED 2. VS 1 hr 3. Keep SpO2 >94% 4. NS 1000 mL bolus over 30 min 5. Cefotaxime 1 g IV piggyback Stat 6. Vancomycin 1 g IV Stat 7. Insert urinary catheter 8. CBC, CMP, urinalysis, urine cultures, sputum cultures, blood cultures, lactate level, PT/PTT, ABG, CXR Stat	1. Initial assessment and evaluation of assessment data 2. Review patient background and current order set 3. Report assessment findings to HCP 4. Administer oxygen 5. Begin IV infusion 6. Insert urinary catheter 7. Administer medications 8. Obtain laboratory or diagnostic test	Provide additional assessment details at learner's request (ie, temperature, weight, laboratory results)
2. Improvement with Fluids	HR = 98 BP = 106/72 RR = 24 SpO2 = 98% on 6 LPM nasal cannula Breath sounds = clear Cardiac rhythm = sinus tachycardia, no ectopy Urine output = 25 mL/h dark gold, cloudy Moans to painful stimuli Temperature = 36.0°C	1. Admit to ICU 2. Central venous access, monitor CVP, PAP, CO, SVR 3. IV 0.9% NS at 160 mL/h until CVP >8 mm Hg, Consult health care provider for further orders when CVP >8 mm Hg 4. Consult surgical resident for arterial catheter placement 5. Call for systolic BP >180 or <100	1. Reassess patient condition and status 2. Interpret assessment findings and documents 3. Monitor the infusion frequently 4. Obtain and interpret laboratory and radiograph results 5. Prepare patient for admission to ICU 6. Give report to ICU RN	Provide additional orders after learners call with assessment and results

(continued on next page)

Table 1
(continued)

State Description	Events or Simulator Actions	Health Care Provider Orders	Learner Expected Behaviors	Faculty Activities
3. Deterioration After Admit to ICU	HR = 144 BP = 68/42 RR = 28 SpO2 = 60% on 6 L/NC Breath sounds = rales Cardiac rhythm = sinus tachycardia Urine output = 10 mL/h dark gold, cloudy No response to painful stimuli	1. Intubate patient 2. Ventilator settings: Vt 600 mL, RR 24, mode AC, PEEP 5, Fio$_2$ 100% 3. Insert Salem sump nasogastric tube and place to low wall suction 4. Portable chest radiograph STAT for endotracheal tube placement 5. Repeat ABG in 30 min	1. Reassess patient, interpret findings, and document appropriately 2. Notify health care provider of significant changes 3. Recognize need for intubation and mechanical ventilation 4. Place head of bed down	Provide additional orders after learners call with assessment and changes in status
4. Code Blue, Multiple Organ System Dysfunction	Sinus tachycardia progresses rapidly to unstable V-Tach with PVCs to V-Fib with CPR in progress then ROSC Remains intubated	1. Arterial line placement 2. ABG Stat	1. Institute Code Blue protocol; each team member has a specific role (team leader, compressions, airway, medications or IV, recorder) 2. Begin CPR on discovery of arrest 3. Safely defibrillate and evaluate response 4. Provide bag-valve ventilations 5. Ensure documentation of activities 6. Support family members on arrival	With the patient stabilizing, the faculty announces the learner's shift is ended

Abbreviations: BP, blood pressure; CBC, complete blood count; CPR, cardiopulmonary resuscitation; CT, computed tomography; ED, emergency department; HR, heart rate; ICU, intensive care unit; IV, intravenous; RN, registered nurse; RR, respiratory rate.

Table 2
Abridged pediatric postoperative sepsis high-fidelity human patient simulation scenario

State Description	Events or Simulator Actions	Health Care Provider Orders	Learner Expected Behaviors	Faculty Activities
1. ED Assessment (baseline)	HR = 110 BP = 115/73 RR = 26 SpO2 = 98% on room air Urine output = 20 mL voided in urinal dark, amber Weight = 25 kg Temperature = 38.4°C Hypoactive bowel sounds with rebound tenderness to abdomen Pain 5/5 on FACES scale	1. Admit to ED 2. VS 3. IV bolus 0.9% NS 20 mL/kg 4. npo 5. CBC, CMP, urinalysis 6. Focused appendiceal CT 7. Acetaminophen supp 10 mg/kg PR q 4 h prn pain or temp >38.4°C	1. Complete initial assessment and include focused abdominal assessment 2. Evaluate pain using appropriate pain rating scale 3. Administer acetaminophen for pain or fever 4. Identify developmentally appropriate interventions to assist patient and family in coping with pain and anxiety 5. Report assessment findings to HCP 6. Begin IV infusion 7. Request and interpret laboratory results 8. Notify radiology of CT order	Provide additional assessment details at learner's request (ie, temperature, complaints of nausea, laboratory results)
2. Rupture of Appendix	HR = 108 BP = 102/68 RR = 24 SpO2 = 98% Breath sounds = clear Temperature = 36.0°C Appears more comfortable sleeping intermittently Pain 1/5 on FACES scale	1. Place nasogastric tube to low wall suction 2. Preoperative dose of ampicillin 200 mg/kg/d IV q 6 h 3. Notify health care provider if temperature >39°C, HR >115, RR >30, BP systolic <100 4. Prepare patient for emergency appendectomy	1. Reassess patient condition and status 2. Interpret assessment findings and documents 3. Obtain and interpret laboratory and radiograph results 4. Prepare patient for transfer to OR or admission to ICU 5. Give report to ICU RN	Provide additional orders after learners call with assessment and results

(continued on next page)

Table 2
(continued)

State Description	Events or Simulator Actions	Health Care Provider Orders	Learner Expected Behaviors	Faculty Activities
3. PICU Postoperative Day 1: Early Sepsis Syndrome	HR = 124 BP = 115/55 RR = 32 SpO2 = 96% Breath sounds = clear Urine output = 50 mL Lethargic Bounding pulses Pain 3/5 Temperature 39.4°C Skin flush and warm	1. Morphine PCA pump basal rate 0.02 mg/kg/h, bolus 0.02 mg/kg, maximum attempts 10/h, lockout 6 min 2. Reinforce dressing prn for first 24 h, then change prn 3. Oxygen at 2 L/NC to maintain SpO2 >95% 4. Incentive spirometry every 1 h	1. Conduct ongoing assessment, interprets findings, and documents 2. Monitor pain levels and provide adequate pharmacologic and developmentally appropriate non-pharmacological interventions to decrease pain 3. Monitor level of consciousness and neurologic function and reports changes 4. Assess wound for healing and signs of infection	Provide additional orders after learners call with assessment and changes in status
4. Postoperative Day 5: Resolving Sepsis and Discharge	HR = 108 BP = 115/73 RR = 20 SpO2 = 99% Breath sounds = clear Awake, alert, Oriented X3 Pain 0/5, Temperature = 37.4°C Interactive, ambulatory and participating in care	1. Discharge to home 2. Diet regular 3. Acetaminophen 325 mg po every 4-6 h as needed for pain 4. Call to schedule follow-up appointment in surgery clinic	1. Conduct ongoing assessment, interpret findings, and document 2. Provide age-appropriate diversional activities 3. Provide developmentally appropriate discharge instructions to patient and family	With the patient discharge, the faculty announces the conclusion of this simulation

FACES refers to the Wong-Baker FACES Pain Rating Scale. A series of faces are shown from a happy face at 0 5 no pain to a crying face or 10 5 hurts the worst.
Abbreviations: 6LPM, 6 liters per minute; ABG, arterial blood gas; AC; assist control; CO, cardiac output; CMP, Comprehensive Metabolic Panel; CVP, central venous pressure; CXR, chest x-ray; FiO2; Fraction of inspired oxygen; HCP, healthcare provider; L/NC, liters per nasal cannula; NS, normal saline; OR, operating room; PAP, pulmonary artery pressure; PCA, patient-controlled analgesia; PEEP; positive end-expiratory pressure; PICU, Pediatric ICU; PR, per rectum; PT/PTT, prothrombin time/partial thromboplastin time; PVCs, Premature ventricular contractions; SpO2, peripheral capillary oxygen saturation; sup, suppository; SVR, Systemic vascular resistance; VS, vital signs; Vt, tidal volume; ROSC, Return of spontaneous circulation; V-fib, ventricular fibrillation; V-Tach, ventricular tachycardia; X3, times.

can feed and toilet himself. He recently received urinary tract infection treatment and completed a course of antibiotics at the nursing home. Mr Smith is now being seen in the emergency department due to increasing unresponsiveness over the past 24 hours. He only responds to painful stimuli by groaning. He has spontaneous eye opening but is unable to follow commands. Additionally, Mr Smith's blood pressure has dropped to the low 100s over 60s, his skin is flushed and cool, and his respirations are slightly labored at 26 breaths per minute. **Table 1** includes an abridged adult sepsis, septic shock HF-HPSim Scenario.

The second example involves the care of Billy, an 8-year-old boy, who has postoperative sepsis due to a ruptured appendix. The patient has been brought to the pediatric emergency department by his parents with signs and symptoms of appendicitis. Billy has been complaining of severe localized pain to the lower right quadrant of the abdomen, nausea, vomiting, and fever. Symptoms began 2 days ago and his mother reports, "He is not acting like himself." He has a loss of appetite over the past 2 days and only ate crackers and a few sips of lemon-lime soda this morning. He has no significant past medical history and never been hospitalized. **Table 2** includes an abridged pediatric postoperative sepsis HF-HPSim scenario.

SUMMARY

Sepsis, including severe and septic shock, is a worldwide health condition with high mortality rates. Nurses are directly involved with the care of patients with a diagnosis of adult or pediatric sepsis. To improve the outcomes of patients with sepsis, nurses must be able to deliver safe, evidence-based care. HF-HPSim can provide an experiential and safe learning environment for nurses to improve confidence, critical thinking, and build on knowledge surrounding care of the patient with sepsis.[21,23,25]

REFERENCES

1. Kleinpell R, Aitken L, Schorr CA. Implications of the new international sepsis guidelines for nursing care. Am J Crit Care 2013;22(3):212–22.
2. Kleinpell RM, Schorr CA, Balk RA. The new sepsis definitions: implications for critical care practitioners. Am J Crit Care 2016;25(5):457–64.
3. Singer M, Deutschmann CS, Seymour CW, et al. The third international consensus definitions for sepsis and septic shock. JAMA 2016;315:801–10.
4. Jeffries PR. Clinical simulations in nursing education: advanced concepts, trends, and opportunities. New York: National League for Nursing; 2014.
5. Cato ML. Using simulation in nursing education. In: Jeffries PR, editor. Simulation in nursing education: from conceptualization to evaluation. New York: National League for Nursing; 2012. p. 1–12.
6. Hayden J. Use of simulation in nursing education: national survey results. J Nurs Regul 2010;1(3):52–7.
7. Nehring WM, Lashley FR. Current use and opinions regarding human patient simulators in nursing education: an international survey. Nurs Educ Perspect 2004; 25:244–8.
8. Jeffries PR, Rogers KL. Theoretical framework for simulation design. In: Jeffries PR, editor. Simulation in nursing education: from conceptualization to evaluation. New York: National League for Nursing; 2012. p. 25–41.
9. Horsley TL, Wambach K. Effect of nursing faculty presence on students' anxiety, self-confidence, and clinical performance during a clinical simulation experience. Clin Simul Nurs 2015;11(1):4–10.

10. Jeffries PR, Swoboda SM, Akintade B. Teaching and learning using simulation. In: Billings DM, Halstead JA, editors. Teaching in nursing: a guide for faculty. St Louis (MO): Elsevier; 2016. p. 304–23.

11. Kolb DA. Experiential learning. Upper Saddle River (NJ): Prentice-Hall; 1984.

12. Anderson JM, Warren JB. Using simulation to enhance the acquisition and retention of clinical skills in neonatology. Sem Perinatol 2011;35:59–67.

13. Cant RP, Cooper SJ. Simulation-based learning in nurse education: systematic review. J Adv Nurs 2009;66(1):3–15.

14. Fabro K, Schaffer M, Scharton J. The development, implementation, and evaluation of an end-of-life simulation experience for baccalaureate nursing students. Nurs Ed Persp 2014;35(1):19–25.

15. Guhde J. Nursing students' perceptions of the effect of critical thinking, assessment, and learning satisfaction in a simple versus complex high-fidelity simulation scenarios. J Nurs Ed 2011;50:73–8.

16. Kaddoura MA. New graduate nurses' perceptions of the effects of clinical simulation on their clinical thinking, learning, and confidence. J Contin Educ Nurs 2010;41(11):506–16.

17. Lancaster RJ. Serious game simulation as a teaching strategy in pharmacology. Clin Sim Nurs 2014;10:e129–37.

18. Lasater K. High fidelity simulation and the development of clinical judgment: students' experiences. J Nurs Ed 2007;46(6):269–76.

19. Przybyl H, Androwich I, Evans J. Using high-fidelity simulation to assess knowledge, skills, and attitudes in nurses performing CRRT. Neph Nurs J 2015;42:135–47.

20. Shin H, Sok S, Hyun KS, et al. Competency and active learning program in undergraduate nursing education. J Adv Nurs 2014;71(3):591–8.

21. Swenty CF, Eggleston BM. The evaluation of simulation in a baccalaureate nursing program. Clin Sim Nurs 2011;7:e181–7.

22. Jeffries PR, Clochesy JM. Clinical simulations: an experiential, student-centered pedagogical approach. In: Billings D, Halstead J, editors. Teaching in nursing: a guide for faculty. St Louis (MO): Elsevier; 2012. p. 352–68.

23. Weaver A. The effect of a model demonstration during debriefing on students' clinical judgment, self-confidence, and satisfaction during a simulated learning experience. Clin Sim Nurs 2015;11:20–6.

24. American Association of Colleges of Nursing. The essentials of baccalaureate education for professional nursing practice. 2008. Available at: http://www.aacnnursing.org/Portals/42/Publications/BaccEssentials08.pdf. Accessed January 3, 2018.

25. Twibell R, St. Pierre J, Johnson D, et al. Tripping over the welcome mat: why new nurses don't stay and what the evidence says we can do about it. Am Nurse Today 2012;7(8):1.

26. Bridges E, McNeill MM, Munro N. Research in review: advancing critical care practice. Am J Crit Care 2017;26(1):77–88.

27. Hovancsek MT. Using simulation in nursing education. In: Jeffries PR, editor. Simulation in nursing education: from conceptualization to evaluation. New York: National League for Nursing; 2007. p. 1–9.

28. Aschenbrenner DS, Milgrom LB, Settles J. Designing simulation scenarios to promote learning. In: Jeffries PR, editor. Simulation in nursing education: from conceptualization to evaluation. New York: National League for Nursing; 2012. p. 43–76.

29. Jeffries PR, Rodgers B, Adamson K. NLN Jeffries simulation theory: brief narrative description. Nurs Ed Persp 2015;36(5):292–3.
30. Decker S, Fey M, Sideras S, et al. Standards of best practices: simulation standard VI: the debriefing process. Clin Sim Nurs 2013;9:e26–9.
31. Husebo SE, O'Regan S, Nestel D. Reflective practice and its role in simulation. Clin Sim Nurs 2015;11:368–75.

Cardiogenic Shock in the Septic Patient
Early Identification and Evidence-Based Management

Todd Tartavoulle, DNS, APRN, CNS-BC[a],*,
Leanne Fowler, DNP, MBA, AGACNP-BC, CNE[b]

KEYWORDS

- Cardiogenic shock • Sepsis • Myocardial dysfunction • Sepsis and heart failure

KEY POINTS

- Sepsis is an inflammatory process that results in vasodilation and increased capillary membrane permeability.
- In sepsis, hemodynamic changes occur, including a decrease in systemic vascular resistance and cardiac output.
- Myocardial dysfunction in sepsis includes impaired contractility.
- Rapid diagnosis, prompt supportive treatment, and revascularization of coronary arteries are priorities in cardiogenic shock.

Sepsis and septic shock are medical emergencies that are responsible for 1 in 4 deaths worldwide.[1] Seven in 10 adult patients with sepsis have chronic diseases such as diabetes, cardiovascular disease, heart disease, and cancer.[2] Such chronic diseases contribute to the patient's risk for sepsis and complicate the patient's treatment and recovery. It is reasonable to deduce that the presence of chronic cardiac disease increases the patient's risk for shock and the mortality risk when septic. Therefore, early identification and initiating the most current best practices are crucial to the patient experiencing optimal outcomes.

BACKGROUND

With the evolution of sepsis research, updated definitions for sepsis and septic shock are available. Sepsis is "a life-threatening organ dysfunction caused by a dysregulated

Disclosure: The authors have nothing to disclose.
[a] LSU Health New Orleans School of Nursing, 1900 Gravier Street, Office 4C6, New Orleans, LA 70112, USA; [b] LSU Health New Orleans School of Nursing, 1900 Gravier Street, Office 4A14, New Orleans, LA 70112, USA
* Corresponding author.
E-mail address: ttarta@lsuhsc.edu

Crit Care Nurs Clin N Am 30 (2018) 379–387
https://doi.org/10.1016/j.cnc.2018.05.006
0899-5885/18/Published by Elsevier Inc.

host response to infection."[1] Septic shock is "a subset of sepsis with circulatory and cellular/metabolic dysfunction associated with a higher risk of mortality."[1] Both definitions articulate the severity of illness for a patient with either diagnosis. Patients with sepsis and preexisting cardiac disease, such as heart failure, are more vulnerable to cardiac and hemodynamic decompensation than patients with different comorbidities.[3]

The pathogenesis of sepsis involves myocardial depression early in the disease state, contributing to organ dysfunction and hemodynamic compromise.[4] An ultimate consequence of sepsis-induced myocardial depression and hemodynamic instability in the patient with chronic heart failure is cardiogenic shock. Cardiogenic shock is a low cardiac output (CO) state resulting in life-threatening end-organ hypoperfusion and hypoxia in the setting of adequate vascular volume.[5–7] The septic patient progressing to cardiogenic shock is likely to have higher morbidity and mortality rates.[7] Nurses must be able to identify and adequately manage patients at risk for sepsis-induced cardiogenic shock.

LITERATURE REVIEW

A literature review was performed to isolate evidence-based practices for identifying and managing patients experiencing sepsis-induced cardiogenic shock. The Cumulative Index to Nursing and Allied Health Literature and PubMed databases were searched using the key words: cardiogenic shock, sepsis, myocardial dysfunction, and sepsis and heart failure. The search was refined to filter related research and literature over the past 10 years. Thirty-five articles were found and their abstracts reviewed. Twenty manuscripts were specific to the topic. Of the 20 manuscripts included in the review, 14 were review of the literature, 3 were guidelines, 2 were consensus statements, and 1 was a randomized controlled trial.

Pathophysiology of Sepsis

Sepsis-induced myocardial dysfunction occurs secondary to myocardial injury from the dysregulated systemic release of inflammatory cytokines in response to the infectious toxin and mitochondrial dysfunction secondary to tissue ischemia. These pathophysiologic mechanisms can lead to the development of cardiogenic shock.[8] Cardiogenic shock is a physiologic response to a disease state such as sepsis. The severity of cardiogenic shock in the septic patient directly correlates to the degree of preexisting myocardial dysfunction and sepsis-induced myocardial injury.[9]

Sepsis-Induced Myocardial Dysfunction

Sepsis-induced myocardial dysfunction occurs immediately in response to endotoxins released by the causative microorganisms. Endotoxins injure endothelial cells, subsequently triggering the release of inflammatory immunocompetent chemicals such as cytokines, tumor necrosis factor, and interleukins. The dysregulated release of such inflammatory chemicals results in myocardial depression, vasodilation, increased capillary permeability, and enhanced nitric oxide production. Nitric oxide decreases myofibril response to calcium, causing mitochondrial dysfunction, the downregulation of beta-adrenergic receptors, and further systemic vasodilation. Consequently, mechanisms to maintain adequate CO and tissue perfusion are compromised secondary to myocardial contractile depression, absolute intravascular volume loss to the interstitial space, and relative intravascular volume loss from systemic vasodilation. Diminished oxygen delivery and increased oxygen demand result in an imbalance of oxygen needs for cellular metabolism, resulting in a state of systemic ischemia. Systemic ischemia then causes more endothelial injury, perpetuates the dysregulated inflammatory response and impaired oxygen metabolism of sepsis, and progresses in the patient, incurring organ dysfunction, septic shock, and (potentially) cardiogenic shock.[4]

Myocardial dysfunction during sepsis involves impaired contractility and the exhaustion of compensatory mechanisms of autonomic nervous system aimed to support tissue perfusion. Sympathetic mechanisms of an increased heart rate, increased vascular resistance, and increased sodium and water retention eventually increases oxygen demand, decreases oxygen delivery, and worsens an already impaired cellular metabolism. In the setting of the dysregulated inflammatory response seen in sepsis, compensatory mechanisms are triggered repeatedly by persistent inflammatory chemical release, a perpetual imbalance of oxygen supply and demand, and progressive systemic ischemia and impaired cellular metabolism. An impaired cellular metabolism results in the conversion of cellular respiration from aerobic to anaerobic metabolism, leading to irreversible cellular death.[9]

In addition to the myocardial depression that occurs in response to circulating inflammatory chemicals during sepsis, myocardial cell ischemia propagates poor electrical conduction and depressed contractility.[10] Injury incurred to greater than 40% of the myocardium results in greater pump failure and a state of circulatory shock.[9] Prolonged, uncorrected myocardial ischemia results in cellular death and irreversible necrosis (myocardial infarction).[10]

CIRCULATORY SHOCK

Circulatory shock involves cardiovascular collapse and cardiac failure secondary to a variety of causes.[11] This article discusses shock secondary to sepsis and cardiogenic shock.

Septic Shock Progression to Cardiogenic Shock

Septic shock is the most common form of shock experienced by critically ill patients worldwide. Septic shock is classified as a distributive shock involving a relative and absolute intravascular volume loss.[11] Septic shock is the consequence of untreated or inadequately treated sepsis. This means circulating endotoxins were not eradicated and the dysregulated inflammatory response was not adequately disrupted. Consequently, circulatory shock (cardiovascular collapse and cardiac failure) occurs due to inadequate volume resuscitation and infectious source control.[4] By definition, the cardiovascular collapse and cardiac failure occurring in cardiogenic shock involves the heart's inability to manage blood volume.[7] The factor differentiating septic shock from cardiogenic shock is the patient's volume status.

The pathogenesis of septic shock to cardiogenic shock can occur because of inadequate treatment (volume resuscitation and infectious source control). In patients with inadequate sepsis treatment, sepsis-induced impaired tissue perfusion leads to myocardial ischemia, myocardial dysfunction and/or infarction, and (ultimately) cardiogenic shock. Septic patients who are adequately treated with intravascular volume replacement and infectious source control do not commonly experience cardiogenic shock unless there is preexisting cardiac dysfunction.[7] Septic patients with chronic heart failure and a reduced ejection fraction (HFrEF; <40%) who are receiving protocol-driven volume resuscitation for sepsis are at risk for volume overload and, potentially, cardiogenic shock. Despite the lack of research, one can deduce how circulating myocardial depressant factors, progressive myocardial ischemia, and impaired cellular metabolism of oxygen occurring with sepsis in the patient with preexisting HFrEF propels the patient to the state of cardiogenic shock. One can also deduce that the progression to cardiogenic shock occurs variably, commensurate to the degree of preexisting dysfunction and severity of sepsis.

EARLY IDENTIFICATION OF CARDIOGENIC SHOCK IN THE SEPTIC PATIENT
Clinical Presentation

During cardiogenic shock, there is a decrease in CO with evidence of hypoperfusion in the presence of adequate intravascular volume. Due to ineffective contractility, there is a reduction in systolic blood pressure (less than 90 mm Hg), a decrease in cardiac index (CI <2.2 L/min per m^2), and an elevated left ventricular diastolic pressure that results in a decrease in coronary artery perfusion and a decrease in oxygen delivery to the tissues.[9]

Cardiogenic shock is defined as having a mean systolic blood pressure less than 90 mm Hg for longer than 30 minutes, CI less than 2.2 L/min, pulmonary artery occlusive pressure (PAOP) greater than 15 mm Hg, and/or evidence of tissue hypoperfusion with adequate intravascular volume. Signs and symptoms of cardiogenic shock can be related to a diminished CO or related to venous congestion. The presentation of cardiogenic shock is differentiated by left or right heart failure.[9,12]

With left heart failure, a decrease in CO results in hypoperfusion of organs. A decrease in perfusion to the myocardium results in colicky-type chest pain. Tachycardia and narrow pulse pressure may be present. Extremities may be cool and mottled because blood is shunted from the peripheral circulation to the vital organs. Urine output may be less than 0.5 mL/kg/h. Blood is shunted away from skeletal muscles and lactic acid buildup will occur. A lactic acid level greater than 4 mmol/L may detect organ dysfunction at the cellular level before the patient exhibits a systolic blood pressure less than 90 mm Hg. Neurologic signs and symptoms include apprehension, impatience, and increasing mental deterioration. Hypoperfusion to the gastrointestinal tract can lead to hypoactive bowel sounds, absent bowel sounds, and a paralytic ileus. Poor left ventricular function causes blood to back up into the lungs, causing cardiogenic pulmonary edema and coarse crackles for breath sounds. Hypercapnia and acidosis will be present on arterial blood gases. Dyspnea and tachypnea will develop because of the cardiogenic pulmonary edema. A third sound (S3) summation gallop heart sound will be heard on auscultation.[9]

Signs and symptoms of right heart failure induced by left heart failure include jugular venous congestion, peripheral edema, increased portal hypertension, and hepatomegaly with already present left side manifestations of pulmonary edema and respiratory distress.[9]

Hemodynamic Findings

Invasive monitoring via pulmonary artery catheter and arterial lines are used in assessing hemodynamics. The pulmonary artery catheter measures pressures within the heart, pulmonary artery, and CO. The arterial line provides continuous monitoring of blood pressure.[13]

CO is the amount of blood ejected from the heart each minute. Normal CO is 4 to 8 L/min; however, the value drops significantly in the presence of cardiogenic shock. CI is calculated via an individual's body surface area and is a more accurate way to measure CO. A CI less than 2.2 L/min^2 is found in cardiogenic shock. In cardiogenic shock, compensatory mechanisms kick in as the body increases heart rate and/or stroke volume in an attempt to increase CI. This increase in heart rate is counterproductive because this causes an increase in oxygen demand of an already damaged heart muscle. A faster heart rate reduces diastolic filling time, which negatively impacts CI even further.[12]

Preload is the volume of blood in the ventricle at the end of diastole. The preload of the right side of the heart is reflected via the central venous pressure (CVP) or right atrial pressure. PAOP reflects preload of the left side of the heart. PAOP will be elevated (greater than 15 mm Hg) in cardiogenic shock and CVP may also be elevated (greater than 12 mm Hg).[14]

Afterload is the resistance the left ventricle must overcome to eject blood from the heart. Afterload depends on the competency of the valves and vascular resistance. Systemic vascular resistance is the afterload of the left ventricle and ranges from 800 to 1200 dyne/s/cm[5]. Pulmonary vascular resistance is the afterload of the right ventricle and is less than 250 dyne/s/cm[5]. In cardiogenic shock, systemic vascular resistance and pulmonary vascular resistance may be elevated due to vasoconstriction of the vasculature as a result of sympathetic stimulation.[14]

Mean arterial pressure (MAP) (60–100 mm Hg) is the average pressure in a patient's arteries during 1 cardiac cycle. MAP is a measurement of tissue perfusion to the vital organs. MAP in cardiogenic shock is not adequate to maintain tissue perfusion. CO directly affects MAP. As CO decreases, so does MAP. Contractility is the force and velocity with which the ventricles eject blood. Contractility can be measured indirectly by the right and left ventricle stroke indexes. In cardiogenic shock there is a decrease in contractility causing a decrease in stroke volume. **Box 1** is a hemodynamic profile of a patient in cardiogenic shock.

Workup

Cardiogenic shock is a medical emergency; therefore, rapid diagnosis, prompt supportive therapy, and expeditious revascularization of coronary arteries in patients with myocardial ischemia and infarction is a priority. A complete workup includes laboratory studies, imaging studies, and invasive hemodynamic monitoring. A complete laboratory workup includes a complete blood count (CBC), cardiac enzymes, arterial blood gases, lactate level, and brain natriuretic peptide (BNP). A biochemical profile includes electrolytes, renal function, and liver function tests, and is collected to assess and monitor the function of vital organs. A CBC will rule out anemia. An elevated white blood cell count may indicate sepsis. Cardiac enzymes, creatine kinase, troponin, myoglobin, and Lactate Dehydrogenase aid in the diagnosis of acute myocardial infarction. Released during myocardial cell injury, troponin I and troponin T are elevated in septic shock and indicate damage to the myocardium. Arterial blood gas values indicate

---

Box 1
Hemodynamic profile for a patient in cardiogenic shock

Normal Value	Cardiogenic Shock Value
Heart rate 60–100 beats per minute (bpm)	>110 bpm
CVP 2–8 mm Hg	>12 mm Hg
Pulmonary artery occlusive pressure 8–12 mm Hg	>15 mm Hg
Systemic vascular resistance 800–1200 dyne/s/cm^5	>1200 dyne/s/cm^5
Pulmonary vascular resistance <200 dyne/s/cm^5	>250 dyne/s/cm^5
CO 4–8 L/min	<4 L/min
CI 2.5–4 L/min	<2.2 L/min
MAP 60–110 mm Hg	<60 mm Hg

Data from Dahling M. Cardiogenic shock and hemodynamic support a realistic management approach. Cath Lab Digest 2003;11(11):1–4.

acid-base balance and arterial oxygen saturation. An elevated serum lactate level indicates organ hypoperfusion and shock. Elevated BNP indicates heart failure.[15]

An echocardiogram, an imaging study, should be performed early to determine the cause of cardiogenic shock. Information on diastolic and systolic function, akinetic or dyskinetic areas of myocardium, ejection fraction, and valve function is revealed with the echocardiogram.[5,16]

Bedside ultrasound can be performed on the inferior vena cava (IVC) to determine fluid status. In a dehydrated patient, the IVC will collapse with respiration. A lack of IVC collapse suggests intravascular euvolemia.[15]

For patients in cardiogenic shock due to myocardial infarction or myocardial ischemia, a 12-lead electrocardiogram (ECG) should be performed. Acute myocardial ischemia is diagnosed by 12-lead ECG based on the presence of ST segment elevation greater than 1.5 to 2 mm, ST segment depression, or Q waves in 2 or more contiguous leads.[15]

EVIDENCE-BASED MANAGEMENT

Initial sepsis therapy includes prompt and broad-spectrum, empiric combination antibiotic therapy in conjunction with surgical removal of the infectious agent, if applicable. Fluid resuscitation with crystalloids of 30 mL/kg should be initiated when the lactate level is equal to or greater than 4 mmol/L, to support the delivery of oxygen and correct hypotension and hypovolemia unless pulmonary edema is present. Mechanical ventilation is frequently required to maintain airway protection and provide oxygenation. Nurses should recognize that positive pressure provided by mechanical ventilation could reduce venous return to the heart.[17]

The overall goal when treating cardiogenic shock is to decrease the workload of the myocardium to allow for cardiac recovery. Optimizing tissue perfusion, restoring of coronary blood flow, improving cardiac function, and controlling infection is imperative. Correction of hypokalemia, hypomagnesemia, and acidosis is also essential.

Central Venous Access and Invasive Monitoring

Placement of a central line and/or pulmonary artery catheter may be helpful in guiding fluid resuscitation and infusing vasoactive agents that are caustic to peripheral vessels. A central venous catheter provides vascular access for multiple infusions concurrently. A pulmonary artery catheter can provide a complete hemodynamic profile, including CO, CI, stroke volume index, and stroke work index. Stroke volume index and stroke work index vary inversely with mortality according to the SHOCK trial. The Surviving Sepsis campaign recommends obtaining a central venous oxygen saturation ($ScVO_2$) greater than 70%. $ScVO_2$ can be obtained via a central venous catheter.[1]

Volume Status Assessment

Assessing volume status via CVP and central line can be difficult and unreliable. More reliable tests, such as IVC compressibility, pulse pressure variation, or other dynamic volume responsiveness indices, may be performed. An arterial line should be placed to most accurately and continuously monitor blood pressure. Continuous arterial blood pressure monitoring is necessary for the accurate titration and evaluation of vasoactive agents used to treat and hemodynamically support the cardiogenic shock patient.[17]

Vasoactive Pharmacotherapeutic Circulatory Support

Vasopressor therapy is recommended when the patient is not responsive to fluid volume resuscitation. Norepinephrine is an alpha-adrenergic agonist and is a first-line vasopressor in septic shock and sepsis-induced cardiac dysfunction.[7] Norepinephrine has minor beta 1-adrenergic agonist effects and can moderately increase heart rate and contractility. Because there is a moderate increase in heart rate and contractility, norepinephrine is not considered a first-line therapy in the treatment of sepsis-induced cardiac dysfunction. Dobutamine is the agent of choice to support myocardial suppression in sepsis-related cardiac suppression or shock (see later discussion).[8]

Vasopressin, also named antidiuretic hormone, may also be an effective vasopressor therapy. Low-dose vasopressin is recommended as an adjunctive agent to norepinephrine to either increase MAP or decrease norepinephrine dosage. The use of low-dose vasopressin alone is not recommended.[8]

Epinephrine is an alpha 1, beta 1, and beta 2 agonist. As a result of its beta 1 agonist properties, epinephrine is a potent inotrope and increases MAP by increasing CI, stroke volume, and systemic vascular resistance. Epinephrine can decrease splanchnic blood flow, increase oxygen delivery and consumption, and induce lactic acidosis. Epinephrine is not recommended as first-line therapy to treat sepsis-induced cardiomyopathy.[17]

Levosimendan, a calcium sensitizer, has been used in Europe to increase coronary blood flow. The drug is not approved by the US Food and Drug Administration. The drug's mechanism of action includes increasing the sensitivity of the cardiac myofilament to calcium. Levosimendan is a potent inotrope and causes arterial, venous, and coronary circulation vasodilation. The drug should not be used with vasoconstrictive agents.[15]

As briefly mentioned previously, for patients with a $ScVO_2$ less than 70% and adequate fluid status, dobutamine is recommended as first-line therapy to increase CI. Dobutamine, a beta receptor agonist inotrope, improves myocardial contractility. The mechanism of action of dobutamine includes activation of adenyl cyclase and increasing intracellular cyclic adenosine monophosphate (cAMP) and calcium levels to induce significant positive and mild chronotropic effects. There is also a decrease in afterload (mild peripheral vasodilation). The ultimate effect is an increase in CI.[17]

It has been suggested that inotropic catecholamines, including dobutamine, may stimulate bacterial proliferation and biofilm formation. This may be a factor in the development of intravascular catheter colonization and catheter-related infection. Dobutamine can also have adverse effects in patients with sepsis-induced cardiomyopathy and, therefore, should be used with caution.[17]

Phosphodiesterase inhibitors are positive inotrope agents and increase cAMP concentration in the cardiomyocyte cytosol. These drugs are not recommended for treatment of sepsis-induced cardiogenic shock due to their vasodilatory effects.[17]

No specific drug can reverse sepsis. Initiation of antibiotic therapy and prompt removal of the infectious agent is a priority. Supportive therapy consisting of fluid resuscitation with vasoconstriction and inotropic agents is crucial to preventing tissue hypoxia.[16]

Mechanical Circulatory Support

Using an intraaortic balloon pump (IABP) or other counterpulsation mechanical circulatory support is not discussed in the latest sepsis guidelines. Nevertheless, research related to the use of mechanical circulatory devices such as a balloon pump for patients who require temporary circulatory support is inconclusively discussed in other research.[7,18,19] Although there is evidence supporting the use of an IABP in cytokine-mediated microcirculation dysfunction (sepsis), there is other research, specifically the IABP-SHOCK II trial, stating that there is minimal improvement of outcomes with myocardial infarction–associated cardiogenic shock.[18–20] High-level research is limited in the use of counterpulsation therapies in the sepsis-induced cardiogenic shock patient. Therefore, medical providers must determine its use on an individual case basis, weighing the patients' risks, benefits, and prognostic indicators.[7]

SUMMARY

Sepsis-induced cardiogenic shock is a lethal condition and the management is challenging. Cardiogenic shock in the septic patient involves myocardial systolic and diastolic dysfunction, and requires supportive pharmacotherapy. Nurses should consider that no specific drug can reverse the myocardial dysfunction associated with sepsis. Rapid diagnosis, prompt appropriate antibiotic therapy, aggressive fluid resuscitation, vasopressor administration, infectious source control, expeditious coronary revascularization, and improved contractility is mandatory to achieving a positive outcome. Studies of sepsis-induced cardiogenic shock continue. Future research should focus on the effects of immunometabolic and neuroendocrine factors on cardiomyocytes at the cellular level. This may provide a better understanding of the factors that contribute to sepsis-induced cardiogenic shock, and identify new therapies to improve prognosis.

REFERENCES

1. Rhodes AE, Evans LE, Alhazzani W, et al. Surviving sepsis campaign: international guidelines for management of sepsis and septic shock 2016. Crit Care Med 2017;45(3):486–552.
2. [CDC], C. f. Sepsis: data & reports. Retrieved from: CDC.org. 2017. Available at: https://www.cdc.gov/sepsis/datareports/index.html. Accessed September 25, 2017.
3. Benjamin EJ. Heart disease and stroke statistics—2017 update. Circulation 2017; 35:e146–603.
4. Howell MD. Management of sepsis and septic shock. JAMA 2017;317(8):847–8.
5. Thiele HZ. Intraaortic balloon support for myocardial infarction. N Engl J Med 2012;367:1287–96.
6. Reynolds HR. Cardiogenic shock: current concepts and. Circulation 2008;117: 686–97.
7. van Diepen S, Katz JN, Albert NM, et al. Contemporary management of cardiogenic shock: a scientific statement from the American Heart Association. Circulation 2017;136(16):e232–68.
8. Sato R, Nasu M. A review of sepsis-induced cardiomyopathy. J Intensive Care 2015;3(48):1–7.
9. Warise L. Understanding cardiogenic shock a nursing approach to improve outcomes. Dimens Crit Care Nurs 2015;34(2):67–78.
10. O'Gara PT. 2015 ACC/AHA/SCAI focused update on primary percutaneous coronary intervention for patients with ST-elevated myocardial infarction. Circulation 2015;133:1135–47.
11. Vincent JL, De Backer D. Circulatory shock. N Engl J Med 2013;369:1726–34.
12. Gorman D, Calhoun K, Carassco M, et al. Take a rapid treatment approach to cardiogenic shock. Nursing 2008;3(4):19–27.
13. McAtee M. Cardiogenic shock. Crit Care Nurs Clin North Am 2011;23:607–15.
14. Dahling M. Cardiogenic shock and hemodynamic support a realistic management approach. Cath Lab Dig 2003;11(3):1–4.
15. Ren X. Cardiogenic shock workup. 2017. Available at: http://emedicine.medscape.com/article/152191-workup. Accessed September 25, 2017.

16. Kakihana Y, Ito T, Nakahara M, et al. Sepsis-induced myocardial dysfunction: pathophysiology and management. J Intensive Care 2016;4(22):1–10.
17. Jozwiak M, Persichini R, Monnett X, et al. Management of myocardial depression in severe sepsis. Semin Respir Crit Care Med 2011;32(21):206–14.
18. den Uil CA, Lagrand WK, van der Ent M, et al. Impaired microcirculation predicts poor outcome of patients with acute myocardial infarction complicated by cardiogenic shock. Eur Heart J 2010;31:3032–9.
19. den Uil CA, Maat AP, Lagrand WK, et al. Mechanical circulatory support devices improve tissue perfusion in patients with end-stage heart failure or cardiogenic shock. J Heart Lung Transplant 2009;28:906–11.
20. Thiele H, Zeymer U, Neumann FJ, et al, IABPSHOCK II Trial Investigators. Intra-aortic balloon support for myocardial infarction with cardiogenic shock. N Engl J Med 2012;367:1287–96.

Hospital Costs Associated with Sepsis Compared with Other Medical Conditions

Denise M. Danna, DNS, RN, CNE*

KEYWORDS

- Surviving sepsis campaign • Sepsis • Septicemia • Sepsis costs
- Hospital-acquired infections

KEY POINTS

- Sepsis affects millions of people annually, resulting in significant mortality. Sepsis is among the costliest conditions for hospital admissions and readmissions. Compared with the top 4 conditions (acute myocardial infarction, congestive heart failure, pneumonia, and chronic obstructive pulmonary disease) that are monitored by the Hospital Readmission Reduction Program, sepsis remains the costliest condition.
- The Surviving Sepsis Campaign's aim is to decrease the morbidity and mortality of patients by the use of a set of guidelines. These guidelines are in a form of 3-hour and 6-hour bundles that focus on improving quality outcomes for patients with a sepsis condition.
- Various resources are available for health care providers when caring for patients with a sepsis condition. These resources include the sepsis or septic shock bundles, the Severe Sepsis Practice Alert by the American Association of Critical-Care Nurses, and the Agency for Healthcare Research and Quality (AHRQ) Quality Toolkit.

INTRODUCTION

Health care costs, access, and population health outcomes have been a priority for policy makers and regulators for years. Health care spending is a large component of the US gross domestic product, reaching 17.9% in 2016 compared with 17.7 in 2015.[1,2] Furthermore, hospital care expenses are the largest component of health care costs, increasing 4.3% beyond spending in 2015, equaling 3.3 trillion dollars in 2016.[1,2] Over the years, hospital-acquired infections (HAIs) have been a focus and continue to be a concern for health care organizations owing to the associated costs, mortality, and morbidity rates.[3] Another condition, sepsis, has caught the attention of

Disclosure Statement: The author has nothing to disclose.
University Medical Center New Orleans, 2000 Canal Street, New Orleans, LA 70112, USA
* 4432 Ithaca Street, Metairie, LA 70006.
E-mail address: Denise.danna@lcmchealth.org

hospitals, insurers, regulatory agencies, and medical providers, and has become a major focus for hospitals. This focus is due to increased hospital costs and mortality, which are due to intensive care treatment and hospital readmissions of patients with sepsis conditions. This article compares the hospital costs for patients with sepsis conditions compared with other medical conditions.

Sepsis

Sepsis is among the chief reasons for increased health care costs, hospital readmission rates, and deaths in the United States. Annually, more than 1.5 million people are diagnosed with this condition, 250,000 people die from sepsis, and 1 in 3 deaths in hospitals is attributed to sepsis.[4] More than 1.8 million emergency room visits were due to sepsis from 2009 to 2011.[4,5] In April 2015, the Centers for Medicare & Medicaid Services (CMS) announced a new program for inpatient hospital reporting to improve the outcomes of patients with sepsis conditions.[6] The *Early Management Bundle, Severe Sepsis/Septic Shock (SEP-1)*, states the sepsis measures that hospitals have been required to report since October 1, 2015.[6] Agencies, including the Agency for Healthcare Research and Quality (AHRQ) and the National Quality Forum (NQF), have developed measures to monitor the outcomes of sepsis. The AHRQ developed the Patient Safety Indicator #13 (PSI 13) Postoperative Sepsis Rate as a provider-level patient safety indicator, which was adopted by the CMS as a composite measure of patient safety.[7] In 2017, the NQF bundle for managing severe sepsis and septic shock (measure 0500) was included in the hospital inpatient quality reporting program.[8] With the addition of these measures, it becomes apparent how widespread, serious, and costly sepsis is for the health care system. Important infection control practices, such as handwashing, decrease infections and possibly sepsis. The CDC reported that higher than 90% of adults and 70% of children who are diagnosed with sepsis presented with an underlying condition that may put them at risk, including specific infections.[4] Sepsis, lung, urinary tract, gut and skin (https://www.cdc.gov/vitalsigns/sepsis/).[4]

Definition of Sepsis

Initially, sepsis was described as a systematic host reaction to an infection.[9] Early in the 1970s, it was described as a type of blood poisoning.[10] In 1992, the American College of Chest Physicians and Society of Critical Care Medicine (SCCM) jointly published a definition of sepsis, which was revisited in 2001.[11] In 2014, the European Society of Intensive Care Medicine and the SCCM met to reassess the definition of sepsis.[12] Sepsis was defined as a "life-threatening organ dysfunction caused by a dysregulated host response to infection."[12(p804)] The task force also reassessed the definition of septic shock, now defined as "a subset of sepsis in which underlying circulatory and cellular metabolism abnormalities are profound enough to substantially increase mortality."[12(p806)] The new definitions are designated as Sepsis-3, noting that the previous definitions used Sepsis-1 (1991) and Sepsis-2 (2001).[12]

Impact of Sepsis: Quality and Costs

The prevalence and incidence of sepsis varies between studies owing to various definitions, various types and causes, and individualized patient factors, such as age, comorbid conditions, race, ethnicity, and gender.[13–16] Men have a higher rate than women, but Nonwhite have a higher incident of sepsis among nonwhite persons compared to white persons.[14–18] It is known that many patients who die from infections will eventually die with sepsis and organ dysfunction.[10] Martin[10] commented that as researchers and physicians gain knowledge about the causes of sepsis, the likelihood increases that a better understanding of the epidemiology of sepsis will occur, improving the overall outcomes.

In *"Incidence and Trends of Sepsis in US Hospitals Using Clinical vs Claims Data, 2009–2014,"* the investigators conducted a retrospective cohort study of 409 academic, community, and federal hospitals.[19] They concluded that there was no noteworthy change in the incidence of sepsis during the study period; however, hospital mortality from sepsis decreased during this time.[19]

The exact cost of health care dollars related to sepsis is difficult to determine owing to various factors. In a systematic review, Arefian and colleagues[13] reported on the costs of sepsis in 37 selected studies that met the eligibility criteria. The eligibility criteria were that the studies were published between January 2005 and June 2015, the cost and analyses were specified, sepsis was defined, and how the costs were calculated was described.[13] The median cost of sepsis was $32,421 and the median cost for the intensive care unit (ICU) admission was $27,461. They concluded that the costs of treating patients with sepsis depended on how the costs were calculated, which differed between health care organizations and geographic regions, as well as the type of sepsis and the population included in the study.[13] One important point was that most patients with sepsis received care in an ICU.

Sepsis is a common reason for admissions and mortalities in the ICU.[20,21] Burchardi and Schneider[22] examined the cost of intensive care treatment of patients with sepsis. They concluded that the high percentage of fixed costs resulted in higher overall cost of patients being cared for in the ICU, mainly due to overhead expenses and the extensive patient length of stay.[22]

Several Healthcare Cost and Utilization Project (HCUP) Statistical Briefs provided data on hospital inpatient and emergency department cost, procedures, diagnoses, and other relevant data. In *National Inpatient Hospital Costs: The Most Expensive Conditions by Payer, 2011: Statistical Brief #160,*[23] sepsis was identified as the most expensive diagnosis for hospitalizations in 2011. It remained so in 2013, as reported in *National Inpatient Hospital Costs: The Most Expensive Conditions by Payer: Statistical Brief #204.*[24]

Table 1 displays the most expensive conditions in US hospitals in 2013 for all payers (ie, Medicare, Medicaid, private insurers, and uninsured patients) and breaks down the costs according to each payer, which accounts for 35.6 million inpatient stays and $381 billion in health care costs.[25] The cost of sepsis for all hospitalizations totaled $23.7 billion, which is 6.2% of the aggregate costs for all hospitalizations, and ranked fourth as the costliest condition across all 4 payers.[24] The mean expense for a patient with a sepsis diagnosis admitted to a hospital was more than $18,000 in 2013, 70% more than other average admissions.[24] Several reasons that sepsis is costly are related to hospital readmissions and ICU services. Torio and Moore[24] indicated that the 20 most expensive conditions accounted for 43.7% of all hospitalizations. Hospital expenses have remained stable but the costs for sepsis increased by 19% from 2011 to 2013, twice as much as other conditions.

In conclusion, across all 4 payer groups, sepsis was the costliest condition compared with the top 20 most expensive diagnoses that required hospitalizations in 2013. One of the major reasons for the high cost is related to hospital readmissions of patients with a sepsis condition.[24]

Hospital Readmissions

The Hospital Readmission Reduction Program (HRRP), a component of the Patient Protection and Affordable Care Act of 2010, was enacted to improve the outcomes of patients and decrease health care costs for Medicare patients.[26] The CMS started

Table 1
Most expensive conditions treated in hospitals in the United States, 2013 for all payers

Rank	CCS Principal Diagnosis Category	Aggregate Hospital Costs, $ Millions	National Costs, %
1	Septicemia	23,663	6.2
2	Osteoarthritis	16,520	4.3
3	Liveborn	13,287	3.5
4	Complication of device, implant or graft	12,431	3.3
5	Acute myocardial infarction	12,092	3.2
6	Congestive heart failure	10,218	2.7
7	Spondylosis, intervertebral disc disorders, other back problems	10,198	2.7
8	Pneumonia	9501	2.5
9	Coronary atherosclerosis	9003	2.4
10	Acute cerebrovascular disease	8840	2.3
11	Cardiac dysrhythmias	7178	1.9
12	Respiratory failure, insufficiency, arrest (adult)	7077	1.9
13	Complications of surgical procedures or medical care	6079	1.6
14	Rehabilitation care, fitting of prostheses, and adjustment of devices	5373	1.4
15	Mood disorders	5246	1.4
16	Chronic obstructive pulmonary disease and bronchiectasis	5182	1.4
17	Heart valve disorders	5151	1.4
18	Diabetes mellitus with complications	5142	1.3
19	Fracture of neck of femur (hip)	4861	1.3
20	Biliary tract disease	4722	1.2
Total for top 20 conditions		181,762	47.7
Total for all stays		381,439	100.0

Abbreviation: CCS, Clinical Classification Software.
From Torino C, Moore B. National inpatient hospital costs: The most expensive conditions by payer, 2013: statistical brief #204. Agency for Healthcare Research and Quality. Available at: http://www.hcup-us.ahrq.gov/reports/statbriefs/sb204-Most-Expensive-Hospital-Conditions.pdf.

this program because no significant decrease in the Medicare 30-day readmission rates occurred between the years of 2004 and 2009.[27] Since 2013, using claims-based data, hospitals have been penalized for the number of unnecessary hospital readmissions for the following diagnoses: acute myocardial infarction (AMI), congestive heart failure (CHF), and pneumonia.[27] In 2015, the HRRP expanded its program to include penalties for hospital readmissions for chronic obstructive pulmonary disease (COPD) and hip and knee replacements because of the high volume and costs of these diagnoses.[28] The CMS uses 30-day readmissions rates to measure quality of care and to guide the pay-for-performance program. Unnecessary readmissions are measured by the hospital's readmission rates, which are adjusted for age, sex, and coexisting conditions. This information is compared with national averages. A preestablished maximum penalty is assessed to the hospital; the penalty is the percentage of the total Medicare payments made to the hospital.[29] The pay-for-performance program has encouraged heath care organizations to identify opportunities for improvements using evidence-based interventions and to improve the patient outcomes focusing on these diagnoses.

Trends in Septicemia Hospitalizations and Readmissions in Selected HCUP States, 2005 and 2010: Statistical Brief #161 focused on patients from 6 states across the United States who had 2 or more hospital admissions for a diagnosis of septicemia over a 1-year period.[30] During this time, a 32% increase in the rate of septicemia hospitalizations occurred, with 16% of patients being admitted 2 or more times in 1 year for treatment of septicemia. Almost half of the patients who were discharged in 2010 with a diagnosis of septicemia were readmitted to the hospital from a long-care facility.[30]

In *Trends in Hospital Readmissions for Four High-Volume Conditions, 2009–2013: Statistical Brief #196*, Fingar and Washington[28] examined trends for all hospital readmissions. They specifically reviewed the top 4 high-volume diagnoses tracked in the HRRP. Readmission rates were (1) AMI (14.7 per 100 index days), (2) CHF (23.5 per 100 index days), (3) COPD (20.0 per 100 index days), and (4) pneumonia (15.5 per 100 index days). These 4 conditions were credited for 13% of all hospital readmissions (500,000) and for overall hospital costs of 7 billion dollars in 2013.[28] Septicemia readmissions were reported as 18.9 per 100 index days.[28]

A Comparison of All-Cause 7-Day and 30-Day Readmissions, 2014: Statistical Brief #230, by Fingar and colleagues,[31] described data on all-cause 7-day readmissions compared with all-cause 30-day readmissions. They defined readmissions as hospitalizations for all causes, including planned and unplanned. Septicemia was listed among the top 20 diagnoses with the highest 7-day and 30-day readmission rates in 2014. The investigators compared schizophrenia and other psychotic disorders and CHF with sepsis hospital readmissions. They noted that CHF and schizophrenia and other psychotic disorders are chronic conditions and were among the top 3 diagnoses with 7-day and 30-day readmissions.[31] Septicemia and schizophrenia and other psychotic disorders had a higher percentage of 30-day readmissions that occurred within 7-days compared with CHF.[31] Overall, due to the larger volume of patients with a diagnosis of septicemia, it was among the top 20 diagnoses with the highest 7-day and 30-day readmission rates compared with other major diagnoses.[31]

A study conducted by Chang and colleagues[32] examined the cost, frequency, and risk factors for patients with sepsis who were readmitted in 30 days compared with the diagnoses of CHF and AMI. They concluded that sepsis was the main contributor to additional costs due to hospital readmissions. The investigators reported that, in the state of California, the projected costs for 30-day readmissions during the study period were $500 million per year for sepsis compared with $229 million per year for CHF and $142 million per year for AMI.[32]

Donnelly and colleagues[33] identified unplanned, all-cause readmissions of sepsis and severe sepsis conditions within 7 and 30 days of discharge using claims-based data. The study conducted a retrospective analysis of 345,657 patients who were discharged with a sepsis diagnosis from hospitals in 2012. They concluded that 1 in 15 patients with severe sepsis was readmitted within 7 days and 1 in 5 patients was readmitted within 30 days of discharge.[33] As noted by other studies, hospital readmissions for sepsis cause a substantial burden on the health care system.

Goodwin and colleagues[34] conducted a study to ascertain the frequency, mortality, cost, and risk factors related to hospital readmission of patients with sepsis to hospitals. The study included 43,452 patients who survived sepsis. The results of the study reported that 26% of the patients were readmitted to the hospital within 30 days and 48% were readmitted within 180 days. The costs were estimated at more than $1.1 billion.[34]

Mayr and colleagues[35] used data from the 2013 Nationwide Readmission Database to determine the readmission rate and cost of sepsis compared with the diagnoses of CHF, pneumonia, AMI, and COPD.[35] The study included hospitalizations from 21 states representing 49% of US inpatients. The investigators concluded that sepsis had a higher 30-day hospital readmission rate (12.2%) compared with CHF (6.7%), pneumonia (5%), COPD (4.6%), and AMI (1.3%).[35] Additional results yielded that the length of stay following hospital readmission was 7.4 days for sepsis compared with 6.7 days for pneumonia, 6.4 days for CHF, 6.0 days for COPD, and 5.7 days for AMI.[35] The estimated mean cost per patient was higher with a sepsis diagnosis ($10,070) compared with pneumonia ($9533), AMI ($9424), CHF ($9051), and COPD ($8417).[35]

In addition to the significant increase in health care costs, hospital readmissions place a strain on the health care system through adverse outcomes such as HAIs, premature discharges, and poor planning for care transition.[27] The 30-day readmission rate is a metric that all hospitals measure and is a priority in hospital quality programs. Sepsis is among the top conditions for hospital readmissions and health care organizations have taken notice.

What Can Hospitals and Healthcare Providers Do to Survive Sepsis?

Most interventions to improve sepsis outcomes have involved protocol-driven approaches. As nurses care for patients with sepsis, the use of evidence-based protocols, engagement in nursing research, and education of patients will result in improvements in patient care, outcomes, and expenses. Nurses can identify patients who are at risk for sepsis, which can result in earlier treatment of these patients.

The AHRQ Quality Toolkit provides recommended best practices for caring for sepsis conditions (eg, postoperative sepsis). The toolkit can be found at https://www.ahrq.gov/sites/default/files/wysiwyg/professionals/systems/hospital/qitoolkit/combined/d4j_combo_psi13-sepsis-bestpractices.pdf. The guidelines include various implementation strategies, such as developing a 1-page screening tool[36,37] and the use of a sepsis resuscitation bundle.[36,38–40] Resources that can be used to reduce sepsis in health care organizations are outlined in the 2017 update from Health Research & Educational Trust.[40] They include a sepsis mortality reduction top 10 checklist, a screening tool, an electronic medical record sepsis screen, a sepsis wall poster, and a sepsis clock.[40] These resources serve as valuable best practices for health care organizations to adopt and customize for their organization.

A resource that was developed by the American Association of Critical-Care Nurses, the Severe Sepsis Practice Alert, is a brief document to guide nurses to improve the management of patients with sepsis. This can be accessed at https://innovations.ahrq.agov/qualitytools/severe-sepsis-practice-alert-and-tools. This tool includes a presentation on sepsis and an audit tool that can be valuable to critical care nurses.

One study examined how to improve patient outcomes with sepsis by using interventions such as early identification of sepsis, timely antibiotic administration, and providing education to health care providers.[41] More than 1000 subjects were included in both the intervention and control periods. Results revealed that there was a 30% decreased chance of patients dying in the intervention period, hospital days were 1.07 less in the ICU, and hospital costs were $1949 less.[41]

In 2004, the Surviving Sepsis Campaign[42,43] initiative started with the objective to decrease mortality and morbidity of patients with sepsis through a set of guidelines, including a sepsis 3-hour resuscitation bundle (**Fig. 1**) and a 6-hour septic shock bundle (**Fig. 2**). In addition, the use of the Surviving Sepsis Campaign guidelines provides potential quality outcomes related to hospital length of stay and mortality in

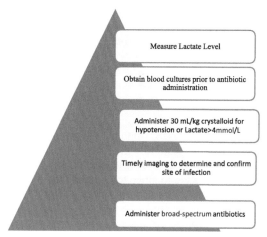

Fig. 1. Sepsis 3-hour resuscitation bundle. (*Reproduced from* survivingsepsis.org; with permission. Copyright © 2015 the Society of Critical Care Medicine and the European Society of Intensive Care Medicine.)

sepsis and septic shock patients. The Surviving Sepsis Campaign resulted in an update of the 2008 guidelines by 68 international experts from more than 30 international organizations.[43]

Recommendations for nursing practice include the implementation of rapid response teams to swiftly respond to critical patient situations, such as patients with sepsis, to decrease preventable deaths.[44] A thorough and consistent nursing handoff provides quality patient care and outcomes. Nurses should be knowledgeable about sepsis guidelines and apply the guidelines to everyday practice.

Further research should be conducted to validate the best practices for nurses in providing nursing care for the patient with sepsis. A study conducted by Aitken and

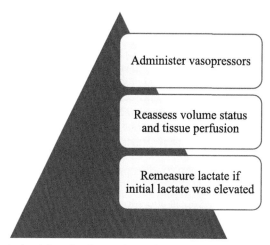

Fig. 2. 6-hour septic shock bundle. (*Reproduced from* survivingsepsis.org; with permission. Copyright © 2015 the Society of Critical Care Medicine and the European Society of Intensive Care Medicine.)

colleagues[45] used a modified Delphi method to provide nurses with 63 recommendations on the best evidence to assist them in caring for patients with sepsis using the Surviving Sepsis Campaign guidelines. The conclusion of the study was that consensus was achieved on many of the recommendations for care; however, further research is needed on several of the recommendations.[45]

SUMMARY

Sepsis is a costly condition that affects millions of patients each year and is among the costliest conditions that affects the US health care system. Increased nursing education focus on the resources available for screening for the signs and symptoms of sepsis, and on the management of patients with sepsis, will be invaluable as hospitals and health care providers continue to strive to decrease the morbidity, mortality, and costs for patients with this life-threatening medical condition.

REFERENCES

1. National Health Expenditures 2016 Highlights. Centers for Medicare & Medicaid Services Web site. 2018. Available at: Reports/NationalHealthExpendData/NationalHealthAccountsHistorical.html2. Accessed January 9, 2018.
2. Hartman M, Martin AB, Espinosa N, et al. National health care spending in 2016: spending and enrollment growth slow after initial coverage expansions. Health Aff (Millwood) 2018;37(1):150–60. Available at: https://www.healthaffairs.org/doi/10.1377/hlthaff.2017.1299. Accessed January 9, 2018.
3. Martin A, Hartman M, Benson J, et al. National health spending in 2014: faster grow driven by coverage expansion and prescription drug spending. Health Aff (Millwood) 2016;35(1):150–60. Available at: http://www.healthaffairs.org/doi/abs/10.1377/hlthaff.2015.1194?journalCode=hlthaff. Accessed January 9, 2018.
4. Data and Reports. Centers for Disease Control and Prevention Web site. 2017. Available at: https://www.cdc.gov/sepsis/datareports/index.html. Accessed January 8, 2018.
5. Wang HE, Jones AR, Donnelly JP. Revised national estimates of ED visits for sepsis in the United States. Crit Care Med 2017;45(9):1443–9.
6. Schorr C. Nurses can help improve outcomes in severe sepsis. Am Nurse Today 2016;11(3):20–5.
7. AHRQ Quality Indicators™ (AHRQI™) ICD-9-CM Specification Version 6.0 Patient Safety Indicator13 (PSI 13) Postoperative Sepsis Rate. Agency for Healthcare Research and Quality Web site. 2017. Available at: https://www.qualityindicators.ahrq.gov/Downloads/Modules/PSI/V60- ICD09/TechSpecs/PSI_13_Postoperative_Sepsis_Rate.pdf. Accessed January 8, 2018.
8. NQF Revises Sepsis Measure. National Quality Forum Web site. Available at: http://www.qualityforum.org/NQF_Revises_Sepsis_Measure.aspx Accessed January 4, 2018.
9. Riedemann N, Guo R, Ward P. The enigma of sepsis. J Clin Invest 2003;112(4): 460–7.
10. Martin G. Sepsis, severe sepsis and septic shock: changes in incidence, pathogens, and outcomes. Expert Rev Anti Infect Ther 2012;1D(6):701–6.
11. American College of Chest Physicians/Society of Critical Care Medicine Consensus Conference: definitions for sepsis and organ failure and guidelines for the use of innovative therapies in sepsis (1992). Crit Care Med 1992;20(6): 864–74.

12. Singer M, Deutschman C, Seymour C, et al. Sepsis definitions task force the third international consensus definitions for sepsis and septic shock (Sepsis-3). JAMA 2016;315(8):801–10.

13. Arefian H, Heublein S, Scherag A, et al. Hospital- related cost of sepsis: a systematic review. J Infect 2016;74(2):107–17.

14. Esper AM, Moss M, Lewis CA, et al. The role of infection and comorbidity: factors that influence disparities in sepsis. Crit Care Med 2006;34(10):2576–82.

15. Martin GS, Mannino DM, Eaton S, et al. The epidemiology of sepsis in the United States from 1979 through 2000. N Engl J Med 2003;348(16):1546–54.

16. Mayr FB, Yende S, Linde-Zwirble WT, et al. Infection rate and acute organ dysfunction risk as explanations for racial differences in severe sepsis. JAMA 2010;303(24):2495–503.

17. Dombrovskiy VY, Martin AA, Sunderram J, et al. Rapid increase in hospitalization and mortality rates for severe sepsis in the United States: a trend analysis from 1993 to 2003. Crit Care Med 2007;35(5):1244–50.

18. Dombrovskiy VY, Martin AA, Sunderram J, et al. Occurrence and outcomes of sepsis: influence of race. Crit Care Med 2007;35(3):763–8.

19. Rhee C, Dantes R, Epstein L, et al. Incidence and trends of sepsis in US hospitals using clinical vs claims data, 2009—2014. JAMA 2017;318(13):1241–9.

20. Genga KR, Russel JA. Update of sepsis in the intensive care unit. J Innate Immun 2017;9(5):441–5.

21. Perner A, Gordon AC, DeBacker D, et al. Sepsis: frontiers in diagnosis, resuscitation and antibiotic therapy. Intensive Care Med 2016;42:1958–69.

22. Burchardi H, Schneider H. Economic aspects of severe sepsis: a review of intensive care unit costs, cost of illness and cost effectiveness of therapy. Pharmacoeconomics 2004;22(12):793–813.

23. Torio C, Andrews R. National inpatient hospital costs: the most expensive conditions by Payer, 2011. HCUP statistical Brief #160. Rockville (MD): Agency for Healthcare Research and Quality; 2013. AHRQ Web site. Available at: https://www.hcup-us.ahrq.gov/reports/statbriefs/sb160.jsp. Accessed January 7, 2018.

24. Torio C, Moore B. National inpatient hospital costs: the most expensive conditions by payer, 2013. HCUP statistical brief #204. Rockville (MD): Agency for Healthcare Research and Quality; 2016. AHRQ Web site. Available at: http://www.hcup-us.ahrq.gov/reports/statbriefs/sb204-Most-Expensive-Hospital-Conditions.pdf. Accessed January 9, 2017.

25. Johnson L, (2017). Expensive Conditions require focus on data and CDI, ICD10 monitor. 2017 Clinical Coding Meeting October 7–8, 2018. Available at: https://www.icd10monitor.com/expensive-conditions-require-focus-on-data-and-cdi. Accessed January 8, 2018.

26. Readmissions reduction program. Centers for Medicare & Medicaid Services Web site. 2017. Available at: https://www.cms.gov/medicare/medicare-fee-for-service-payment/acuteinpatientpps/readmissions- reduction-program.htm. Accessed January 8, 2018.

27. Berenson RA, Paulus RA, Kalman NS. Medicare's readmissions-reduction program – a positive alternative. N Engl J Med 2012;366:1364–6.

28. Fingar K, Washington R. Trends in hospital readmissions for four high-volume conditions, 2009-2013. HCUP Statistical Brief #196. Rockville (MD): Agency for Healthcare Research and Quality; 2015. Available at: http://www.hcup-us.ahrq.gov/reports/statbriefs/sb196-Readmissions-Trends-High- Volume-Conditions.pdf. Accessed January 11, 2018.

29. McIlvennan CK, Eapen ZJ, Allen LA. Hospital readmissions reduction program. Circulation 2015;131:1796–803.
30. Sutton J, Friedman B. Trends in septicemia hospitalizations and readmissions in selected HCUP states, 2005 and 2010. HCUP statistical brief #161. Rockville (MD): Agency for Healthcare Research and Quality; 2013. Available at: http://www.hcup-us.ahrq.gov/reports/statbriefs/sb161.pdf.Updated. Accessed January 10, 2018.
31. Fingar KR, Barrett ML, Jiang HJ. A comparison of all-cause 7-day and 30-day re-admissions, 2014. HCUP statistical brief #230. Rockville (MD): Agency for Health-care Research and Quality; 2017. Available at: hwww.hcup-us.ahrq.gov/reports/statbriefs/sb230-7-Day-Versus-30-Day-Readmissions.jsp. Accessed October 21, 2017.
32. Chang DW, Tseng C-H, Shapiro MF. Rehospitalizations following sepsis: common and costly. Crit Care Med 2015;43(10):2085–93.
33. Donnelly JP, Hohmann SF, Wang HE. Unplanned readmissions after hospitaliza-tion for severe sepsis at academic medical center-affiliated hospitals. Crit Care Med 2015;43(9):1916–27.
34. Goodwin AJ, Rice DA, Simpson KN, et al. Frequency, cost, and risk factors of re-admissions among severe sepsis survivors. Crit Care Med 2015;43(4):738–46.
35. Mayr FB, Talisa VB, Balakumar V, et al. Proportion and cost of unplanned 30-day readmissions after sepsis compared with other medical conditions. JAMA 2017; 317(5):530–1.
36. Dellinger RP, Levy MM, Rhodes A, et al. Surviving the sepsis campaign: interna-tional guidelines for management of severe sepsis and sepsis shock 2012. Crit Care Med 2013;41(2):580–637.
37. Cardoso T, Carneiro AH, Ribeiro O, et al. Reducing mortality in severe sepsis with the implementation of a core 6-hour bundle: results from the Portuguese community-acquired sepsis study (SACiUCI study). Crit Care 2010;4(3):R83.
38. Hospital Inpatient Quality Reporting (IQR) Program measures (calendar year 2014 discharges). (Prepared by Telligen under contract to the Centers for Medi-care & Medicaid Services). Available at: http://www.aqaf.com/perch/resources/library/inpatient-qrdeadlines0911131.pdf. Accessed January 8, 2018.
39. Wang Z, Xiong Y, Schorr C, et al. Impact of sepsis bundle strategy on outcomes of patients suffering from severe sepsis and septic shock in china. J Emerg Med 2013;44(4):735–41.
40. Health Research & Educational Trust [HRET] 2017. Sepsis and septic shock change package. Chicago: Critical Care Medicine; 2017. Health Research & Educational Trust. American Hospital Association Web site. Available at: http://www.hret-hiin.org/. Accessed January 8, 2018.
41. Armen SB, Freer CV, Showalter JS, et al. Improving outcomes in patients with sepsis. Am J Med Qual 2016;31(1):56–63.
42. Surviving Sepsis Campaign. Surviving sepsis. Available at: http://www.survivingsepsis.org/SiteCollectionDocuments/SSC_Bundle.pdf. Accessed January 8, 2018.
43. Kleinpell R, Aitken L, Schorr C. Implications of the new international sepsis guide-lines for nursing care. Am J Crit Care 2013;22(3):212–22.
44. Blont S, Afonso E, Labeau S. Insight and advances in multidisciplinary critical care: a review of recent research. Am J Crit Care 2014;23(1):70–80.
45. Aitken LM, Williams G, Blot S, et al. Nursing considerations to complement the Surviving Sepsis Campaign guidelines. Crit Care Med 2011;39(7):1800–18.

Special Considerations for the Septic Patient Going to the Operating Room

Juanita L. Derouen, DNP, APRN, CRNA*

KEYWORDS

- Sepsis • Septic shock • Perioperative care • Intraoperative care • Intensive care
- Fluid resuscitation • Hemodynamic changes

KEY POINTS

- Perioperative care of the septic patient presents unique challenges for the nurse, such as requiring vigilant assessments and the ability to rapidly address challenging hemodynamic changes.
- Astute critical thinking skills allow the nurse to address the current patient presentation while anticipating potential life-threatening changes that the septic patient may experience.
- The septic patient going to the operating room will benefit from perioperative goal-directed nursing care.

INTRODUCTION

Perioperative care of the septic patient presents unique challenges for nursing care. Because the spectrum of sepsis ranges from early sepsis to septic shock, and because the patient's acuity can change suddenly, nursing care for the septic patient going to the operating room requires an astute eye and vigilant, continuous assessments.

Sepsis causes a dysregulated inflammatory response that leads to hypoperfusion of the body's organs that can progress to multiple organ failure and can ultimately lead to death.[1] Because sepsis is caused by infection, the septic patient may need surgery to eliminate the underlying cause or source of the infection. For example, a patient with an obstructive ureteral calculus may present in urosepsis and need a ureteral stent to relieve the obstruction and allow the kidney to drain and relieve hydronephrosis. Another example would be a patient presenting with an abdominal abscess or bowel perforation that needs surgical intervention to remove the infective source or debride

Disclosure Statement: The author has nothing to disclose.
Department of Anesthesia, Memorial Hospital at Gulfport, 4500 Thirteenth Street, Gulfport, MS 39501, USA
* 23524 Stablewood Circle, Pass Christian, MS 39571.
E-mail address: NitaCRNA45@gmail.com

the infected area. Understanding the physiology of sepsis is important for the nurse to anticipate the physiologic changes associated with the disorder and anticipate the needs of the patient. The nurse has to consider the continuum of sepsis from infection and bacteremia to septic shock when planning the nursing care of a patient going to surgery.[2] Because sepsis causes dysregulation of end-organ perfusion, prompt recognition of increasing severity of the disorder and implementing treatment are needed to prevent degeneration into septic shock.[3] For these reasons a septic patient who is going to surgery will need special considerations preoperative, intraoperative, and postoperative in order to decrease the morbidity and mortality associated with sepsis.

When a surgeon decides to take a septic patient to surgery, they must consider the risks that the stress of the operation will have on the patient as well as the exaggerated hemodynamic changes induced by the anesthetic against the benefits that the procedure will have on the patient. When a patient is critically ill and surgical intervention is necessary to correct the underlying focus of the sepsis, then the decision to go to surgery is often an emergent one because the risk of not doing the surgery outweighs the risks of doing the surgery.[4] Under normal circumstances surgery is planned and the patient is optimized medically. This means that blood pressure, heart rate, blood glucose levels, and other potential system disturbances are addressed and improved before surgery. When a patient is septic and needing surgical intervention emergently, there is no time for optimization and the surgical team will have to care for the patient moment to moment.

PREOPERATIVE CONSIDERATIONS

The septic patient may present in a variety of acuity levels. A patient in early sepsis may be ill in appearance but may be maintaining their airway and showing no difficulty breathing. A patient in early sepsis being prepared for surgery will benefit from oxygen delivered by nasal cannula and should be continuously monitored by pulse oximetry for changes in their respiratory status. A patient going to surgery who has digressed into septic shock may have significantly impaired oxygen exchange and benefit from endotracheal intubation and mechanical ventilation. Regardless of presentation, ensuring adequate airway, breathing, and circulation is the key assessment priority for the nurse.[5]

Prompt administration of preoperative antibiotics is crucial to diminishing the cascade of sepsis.[6,7] The overall goal in caring for the septic patient is elimination of the infection causing the sepsis; however, identification of the cause of infection is not always easy. The infection may be due to Gram-positive or Gram-negative bacteria or may be caused by a fungal infection. Culture negative sepsis occurs in more than half of septic cases where an organism is not identified.[8,9] Often a septic patient presenting for surgery will have blood drawn at the same time that the intravenous (IV) line is placed and blood cultures can be drawn and sent before administration of IV antibiotics. Initiating antibiotics before obtaining cultures can lead to a false-negative result and potentially delay appropriate antibiotic therapy. For this reason, obtaining cultures before antibiotic therapy is important; however, antibiotic therapy should not be delayed waiting on culture results. Antibiotics should ideally be initiated within the first hour of the patient presenting for treatment.[10] Physicians often order broad-spectrum antibiotics be started as soon as possible after obtaining a history in search of potential causes of the infection. In the case of the septic patient who is going to surgery, the source has likely been identified and antibiotic therapy that is likely to eradicate the offending bacteria has been ordered.

Adequate IV access is crucial for fluid resuscitation in the septic patient. Diminishing the hypoperfusion of end organs caused by sepsis is vital and should first be treated with IV fluids. Obtaining at least one large bore IV preoperatively will allow for IV antibiotic therapy to commence and will allow for fluid resuscitation to begin. Two large bore peripheral IVs would be preferred when possible. Peripheral IV access may be adequate for the septic patient going to surgery but central venous access should be considered because of the amount of fluids needed during surgery as well as the potential needed for vasopressors before, during, or after surgery. Extravasation of vasoactive drugs can lead to tissue necrosis, so administration of these drugs through central venous access is the preferred route. Blood products may be needed during the perioperative period as well. Ideally blood products should be infused through a large bore peripheral IV or a central venous access to limit lysis of cells as they are infused. A central venous access catheter also allows for central venous pressures (CVP) to be monitored. The goal of fluid resuscitation is to maintain a CVP of 8 to 12 mm Hg ($\geq$8 mm Hg in a spontaneously breathing patient and $\geq$12 mm Hg in a mechanically ventilated patient). A central venous catheter also allows for monitoring of central venous oxygenation saturation with the goal being greater than 70 mm Hg.[11]

Fluid Resuscitation Goals

- Pulse between 60 and 100 bpm
- Mean arterial pressure 65 to 90 mm Hg
- CVP 8 to 12 mmHg
- Central venous oxygen saturation greater than 70 mm Hg
- Urine output greater than 0.5 cc/kg/h[5,11]

The type of IV fluids ordered will depend on the source of infection and patient presentation. The Surviving Sepsis Campaign 2012 (SSC 2012) recommends crystalloids as the initial resuscitation fluid. Albumin is suggested when large amounts of crystalloids are needed. Colloids will increase oncotic pressure, which decreases fluid shifts in the hours and days that follow. Vasopressors may be used anytime during the perioperative period with the goal of achieving a mean arterial pressure (MAP) of greater than 65 mm Hg. The use of vasopressors is used after adequate fluid replacement. Fluid replacement should occur before the use of vasopressors as a first-line treatment for hypotension in the septic patient; however, in severe sepsis the use of vasopressors may be necessary along with aggressive fluid resuscitation to ensure end-organ perfusion when hypotension is profound. The use of norepinephrine showed a decrease in short-term mortality rates over dopamine in clinical studies. Dopamine has been associated with increased arrhythmias so it is not recommended for first-line treatment of hypotension in the septic patient. For these reasons the recommendations of SSC 2012 are norepinephrine as the first-line choice vasopressor and epinephrine as an alternative to norepinephrine. Vasopressin up to 0.03 to 0.04 unit/min is recommended when the patient does not respond to norepinephrine or epinephrine; however, it is not recommended for use as the only vasopressor. In patients who present with bradycardia, dopamine may be considered.[11]

Vasopressor Therapy Recommendations

- Norepinephrine (first-choice vasopressor)
- Epinephrine (as alternative to norepinephrine)
- Vasopressin in conjunction with norepinephrine or epinephrine
- Dopamine is considered if patient exhibits bradycardia[11]

Preoperative preparation for the septic patient may include insertion and monitoring of an arterial line. The goal of MAP ranges from 65 to 90 mm Hg to ensure end-organ perfusion.[11] An arterial line allows for monitoring of the patient's blood pressure with every beat of the heart versus waiting every few minutes for a noninvasive blood pressure cuff to cycle. The arterial waveform also gives some indication of the fluid/volume status. The dicrotic notch on the arterial waveform represents closure of the aortic valve. Dampening of this waveform, especially in the mechanically ventilated patient, may indicate a decrease in the patient's fluid/volume status.[12] A urinary catheter is placed in these patients to monitor urine output. Fluid resuscitation is guided to maintain a urine output of greater than 0.5 mL/kg/h.[5]

Another consideration worthy of note is mental status evaluation of the awake, spontaneously breathing patient. A change in mental status may indicate decreased brain perfusion and worsening sepsis.[13] The nurse preparing the septic patient for surgery should consider the patient's mental status when obtaining the history as well as the consent for surgery. Having a family member present or a family member's contact information can alleviate delays in getting the patient to surgery if the patient's mental status were to change. If the patient is critically ill and placed on mechanical ventilation, then history may only be able to be obtained from a friend or family member. Trying to establish the last time the patient ate or drank is beneficial for report to the anesthesia staff caring for the patient in the operative arena. This information is also helpful if the patient's respiratory status deteriorates to the point of needing to be intubated before surgery due to the risk of aspiration during endotracheal intubation.[14]

Keeping the patient NPO before surgery is important when possible. If the patient is already intubated this is not a factor, but a spontaneously breathing patient going to surgery preferably needs to be NPO for 6 hours.[14] This decreases the risk of aspiration of gastric contents during manipulation of the airway during endotracheal intubation. The septic patient presents a challenge for the surgical team because these cases are often unscheduled and declared emergent by the surgeon. If a case is judged to be emergent by the surgeon, NPO guidelines are deemed secondary to the emergent need of the surgery and anesthesia personnel use a rapid sequence induction to decrease the risk of aspiration for endotracheal intubation.

INTRAOPERATIVE CONSIDERATIONS

Prompt initiation of IV antibiotic therapy is paramount in caring for the septic patient. Maintaining the schedule of the prescribed antibiotics ensures therapeutic levels of these antimicrobials. Antibiotics that will be due during the time the patient will be in the operating room should be sent with the patient to surgery; however, if a septic patient is going to the operating room there should be no delay in getting the patient to this point of care. Transferring the patient to the operating room should not be delayed while waiting for subsequent antibiotic doses to come from the pharmacy because these can be sent directly to the operating room.

Report for the surgical team should include the following:

- Past medical history
- Medication allergies
- Current vital signs
- Schedule of when the next dose of antibiotic is needed
- Types of IV access (central and/or peripheral access)
- Special monitors (arterial line or central venous access)
- List of any vasoactive or supportive medications

- Intake and output values
- NPO status
- The patient's response to IV fluid resuscitation is also helpful in guiding ongoing fluid replacement therapy

Because these patients often exhibit intraoperative hemodynamic instability, they may require prolonged intubation past the point of surgery. Along with the potential need for extended intubation, the vacillating hemodynamic profile the patient exhibits during surgery may necessitate the continued use of vasopressors and thus require an intensive care unit admission postoperatively.[4] The nurse should anticipate the level of postoperative care needed for the patient. Because these cases are often deemed emergent and can occur after hours, anticipating resources with limited staffing can help ease the transitions from intraoperative to postoperative care.

Special equipment may be needed in the operating room. The nurse needs to consider having point-of-care laboratory testing equipment available in the operating room because this is often helpful during surgery to assess fluid resuscitation. Serial arterial blood gasses and serial lactate testing allow for optimal fluid replacement. Volume resuscitation devices capable of delivering larger fluid volumes may be needed during surgery. The nurse should also prepare for postoperative imaging because the placement of a central venous access may occur after the induction of anesthesia. Portable chest radiographs should be anticipated immediately after surgery to assess positioning of these invasive lines.

POSTOPERATIVE CONSIDERATIONS

Many of these septic surgical patients will require intensive care admissions for their postoperative care. Individuals admitted to intensive care are given the Acute Physiologic and Chronic Health Evaluation score or APACHE score. This is a score that aids in predicting morbidity and mortality in this population of patients.[15] The APACHE IV uses a computerized algorithm using the worst physiologic values measured within 24 hours of intensive care admission. The APACHE score for a postoperative septic patient should use the numeric values derived before resuscitation efforts.[11] The APACHE IV uses 129 variables in its algorithm. The APACHE IV score is shown to be an effective tool in predicting morbidity and mortality in septic patients in clinical studies.[15,16]

Because of the hemodynamic instability of the septic patient, large volumes of fluids are often used in conjunction with vasoactive medications preoperatively and intraoperatively to maximize end-organ perfusion. Prolonged mechanical ventilation may be the safest way to ensure a secure airway and ventilation for these patients after surgery because fluid shifts will begin to occur in the postoperative period. The goal of mechanical ventilation is to minimize prolonged ventilation-induced barotrauma to the lungs. For this reason low-pressure settings are often used along with a high factional inspired oxygen concentration (FiO_2). Tidal volumes of 6 mL/kg decrease the incidence of high-end expiratory pressures and lessen the chance of barotrauma. Hypercapnia is accepted as long as the arterial pH does not drop below 7.2.[17] Fractional inspired oxygen concentration (FiO_2) is titrated to achieve an SpO_2 between 93% and 95%.[11]

Antibiotic therapy is continued in the postoperative period and continuously monitored and adjusted as cultures and sensitivities that were obtained become available. Antibiotic therapy is ideally limited to 7 to 10 days to prevent antibiotic resistance or toxicity.[18]

Depending on the patient's original hematologic profile and the amount of blood that is lost in surgery, blood products may be used during surgery or in any time in the perioperative period. Studies have shown that mortality rates were lower when transfusion was avoided until the patient's hemoglobin was less than 7 g/dL. The exception to this would be a patient with a history of significant coronary artery disease, myocardial infarction, or unstable angina. In high-risk cardiac patients, this permissible anemia does not outweigh the risk of decreased myocardial oxygenation and thus transfusion would need to be initiated at a higher hemoglobin level. Other blood products such as fresh frozen plasma or platelets are needed for bleeding when clotting abnormalities are identified or if large volumes of packed red blood cells have been used. Once concerns of coagulopathy are resolved, deep venous thromboprophylaxis should be considered.[11]

Blood glucose monitoring should be maintained during the entire perioperative period and continued into the postoperative period. In a large randomized trial, there was no significant difference in the outcomes of severely septic patients when strict glycemic and liberal glycemic controls were used. Although outcomes were similar between the 2 groups, there were a greater number of hypoglycemic incidences in the strict glycemic control group. For this reason blood glucose should be maintained between 108 and 180 mg/dL.[19] Nutritional support for these critical patients is imperative to healing. Enteral nutrition by way of nasogastric tube has proved superior over total parenteral nutrition (TPN) in maintaining electrolytes and nutrition; however, TPN may be needed if enteric nutrition is contraindicated in the patient. A patient receiving TPN should continue TPN throughout surgery and the perioperative period to decrease the incidence of hypoglycemia.[20] Keeping in mind that the septic patient who has been to surgery and is now in their recovery phase has received large amounts of fluid, the nurse must be aware that fluid shifts will be occurring in the days following surgery and these shifts can complicate recovery. Congestive heart failure can occur with fluid overload, so frequent auscultation of breath sounds and monitoring for peripheral edema should be included in the nurse's assessment along with CVP values when a central venous access line is available. Serial portable chest radiographs are often ordered to monitor the lung fields for infiltrates and to monitor the size of the cardiac silhouette for signs of cardiac failure and fluid overload. Renal insult is common is septic patients, and acute renal failure occurs in 23% of severely septic patients. Serial laboratory chemistry values such as potassium, blood urea nitrogen, creatinine, glucose levels, and lactate as well as brain natriuretic peptic levels and complete blood counts must be monitored for fluid overload, renal function, and effectiveness of fluid resuscitation. Antimicrobial titers are monitored when indicated as well as a host of other laboratory values depending on the patient's status and comorbidities. Arterial blood gas values are monitored for acid-base levels and effectiveness of oxygen therapy. Current recommendations do not recommend sodium bicarbonate for acidosis unless the pH is <7.1. Hemodialysis may be needed on a temporary basis to aid in recovery from the renal insult brought on by sepsis.[21]

Finally, nurses must remember to consider the families of these patients. It is important to inform the patient's family on the current status of the patient at each stage of perioperative care as well as updating them regularly with any status change. Family members may not understand the importance of invasive lines before surgery. They may not comprehend the urgency of surgery for a family member who is septic and in need of emergent surgical intervention. They should also be told of the potential for prolonged endotracheal intubation and invasive lines in order to know what to expect after surgery. Preparing the family for how they may see their loved one after surgery may make their initial contact with their loved one easier if mechanical ventilation or invasive lines are used. Realistic expectations are often hard to accept by the family so pastoral care or social services may be indicated.

SUMMARY

Nursing care for the septic patient going to the operating room is complicated. Care must be guided by patient presentation and be versatile enough to change with this dynamic illness. Ensuring prompt administration of antibiotic therapy and initiating fluid resuscitation while at the same time ensuring adequate airway and oxygenation is the first step in decreasing the morbidity and mortality of the sepsis cascade. Getting the patient to the operating room in the safest, most expeditious manner allows the surgeon to address the septic foci and eliminate the source of infection. This type of organization and forethought requires astute critical thinking skills. The nurse should know what resources are available to them and anticipate the needs of this patient throughout the perioperative period.

REFERENCES

1. Neviere R. Sepsis syndromes in adults: epidemiology, definitions, clinical presentation, diagnosis, and prognosis. In: Parsons PE, Finlay G, editors. UpToDate. Waltham (MA): UpToDate Inc. Available at: http://www.uptodate.com. Accessed May 15, 2017.
2. Singer M, Deutschman CS, Seymour CW, et al. The third international consensus definitions for sepsis and septic shock (Sepsis-3). JAMA 2016;315(8):801–10.
3. Dellinger RP, Levy MM, Rhodes A, et al. Surviving sepsis campaign: international guidelines for management of severe sepsis and septic shock: 2012. Crit Care Med 2013;41:580–637.
4. Hofer JE, Nunnally ME. Taking the septic patient to the operating room. Anesthesiol Clin 2010;28(1):13–24.
5. Schmidt GA, Mandel J. Evaluation and management of suspected sepsis and septic shock in adults. In: Parsons PE, Sexton DJ, Hockberger RS, et al, editors. UpToDate. Waltham (MA): UpToDate Inc. Available at: http://www.uptodate.com. Accessed July 28, 2017.
6. ProCESS Investigators, Yealy DM, Kellum JA, Huang DT, et al. A randomized trial of protocol-based care for early septic shock. N Engl J Med 2014;370:1683.
7. Zahar JR, Timsit JF, Garrouste-Orgeas M, et al. Outcomes in severe sepsis and patients with septic shock: pathogen species and infection sites are not associated with mortality. Crit Care Med 2011;39:1886.
8. Martin GS, Mannino DM, Eaton S, et al. The epidemiology of sepsis in the United States from 1979 through 2000. N Engl J Med 2003;348:1546.
9. Gupta S, Sakhuga A, Kumar G, et al. Culture-negative severe sepsis: nationwide trends and outcomes. Chest 2016;150:1251.
10. Eissa D, Carton EG, Buggy DJ. Anaesthetic management of patients with severe sepsis. Br J Anaesth 2010;105(6):734–43.
11. Yuki K, Murakami N. Sepsis pathophysiology and anesthetic consideration. Cardiovasc Hematol Disord Drug Targets 2015;15(1):57–69.
12. McGee BH, Bridges EJ. Monitoring arterial blood pressure: what you may not know. Crit Care Nurse 2002;22(2):60–79.
13. Postelnicu R, Evans L. Monitoring of the physical exam in sepsis. Curr Opin Crit Care 2017;23(3):232–6.
14. Yasmin R, Khan SA, Sarker PC, et al. Pre-operative fasting guidelines: an update. Journal of Bangladesh Society of Aenesthesiologists 2009;22(1):32–4.

15. Kelley MA. Predictive scoring systems in the intensive care unit. In: Manaker S, Finlay G, editors. UpToDate. Waltham (MA): UpToDate Inc. Available at: http://www.uptodate.com. Accessed September 19, 2017.

16. Dahhan T, Jamil M, Al-Tarifi A, et al. Validation of the APACHE IV scoring system in patients with severe sepsis and comparison with the APACHE II system. Crit Care 2009;13(Suppl 1):P511.

17. Hager DN, Krishnana JA, Hayden DL, et al. Tidal volume reduction in patients with acute lung injury when plateau pressures are not high. Am J Respir Crit Care Med 2005;172:1241–5.

18. Kumar A. Optimizing antimicrobial therapy in sepsis and septic shock. Crit Care Clin 2009;25:733–51, viii.

19. Brunkhorst FM, Engel C, BLoos F, et al, German Competence Network Sepsis (Sepnet). Intensive insulin therapy and pentastarch resuscitation in severe sepsis. N Engl J Med 2008;358:125–39.

20. Laterre PF, Levy H, Clermont G, et al. Hospital mortality and resource use in sub-groups of the Recombinant Human Activated Protein C Worldwide Evaluation in Sever Sepsis (PROWESS) trial. Crit Care Med 2004;32:2207–18.

21. Shiffle H, Lang SM, Fischer R. Daily hemodialysis and the outcome of acute renal failure. N Engl J Med 2002;346:305–10.

Early Identification and Management of the Septic Patient in the Emergency Department

Jessica Landry, DNP, FNP-BC[a],*,
Leanne H. Fowler, DNP, MBA, AGACNP-BC, CCRN, CNE[b]

KEYWORDS

- Sepsis • Septic shock • Emergency department

KEY POINTS

- Early detection of sepsis in the undifferentiated patient is critical to decrease mortality rates.
- Early antimicrobial treatment is indicated with adequate fluid therapy for best outcomes.
- Goals for treatment include maintaining tissue and organ perfusion while identifying and treating the source.

INTRODUCTION

Sepsis and septic shock affect millions of people around the globe and kills more than 1 in 4 patients worldwide.[1] Emergency departments (EDs) nationwide have implemented evidence-based protocols to facilitate the early detection and treatment of patients with sepsis. Despite these efforts, patients present to the ED undifferentiated and can often have an unclear source of infection. The latest literature provides refined definitions and clinical criteria for sepsis identification and indicates that early detection combined with the appropriate early management improves the septic patients' morbidity and mortality rates.[1-3] ED medical providers have a unique opportunity to improve the septic patient's outcomes when using current clinical practice guidance.[4]

Disclosure: None.
[a] Nursing, Louisiana State University Health, New Orleans School of Nursing, 1900 Gravier Street, Office 161, New Orleans, LA 70114, USA; [b] Adult/Geron Acute Care Nurse Practitioner Program, LSU Health School of Nursing, 154 Islander Drive, Slidell, LA 70458, USA
* Corresponding author.
E-mail address: jland7@lsuhsc.edu

Crit Care Nurs Clin N Am 30 (2018) 407–414
https://doi.org/10.1016/j.cnc.2018.05.009
0899-5885/18/Published by Elsevier Inc.

SEPSIS-3 CLINICAL PRACTICE GUIDANCE
New Definitions

The Sepsis-3 guidelines refined the definitions and categories of sepsis in an effort to connect the diagnoses with the clinical manifestations seen on patient presentation. New definitions shift the focus of sepsis from an infection causing a systemic inflammatory response syndrome (SIRS), such as a bacteremia, to an infection causing SIRS and organ dysfunction (formally called severe sepsis).[2] The most recent sepsis research indicated patients found to have sepsis without organ dysfunction may have experienced iatrogenic volume overload and the overexposure of broad spectrum antibiotics subsequently increasing their morbidity and mortality rates. The shift of focus for the sepsis definition to patients with organ dysfunction captures those patients with the highest risk for death and avoids the potential for the overtreatment of patients with an infection but no evidence of organ dysfunction.[2]

Sepsis is now defined as "life-threatening organ dysfunction caused by a dysregulated host response to infection."[2] Septic shock is now defined as a subset of sepsis involving "circulatory and cellular/metabolic dysfunction that is associated with a higher risk of mortality."[2] The urgency needed in the early identification of sepsis, as it is now defined, exists because of the patient's increased risk for mortality.[1,2]

Clinical Criteria for Sepsis

To screen a large number of undifferentiated patients for sepsis or septic shock, an index of suspicion and valid screening mechanism is required at the time of the patient's arrival.[3] For many years, SIRS criteria have been used in hospital-wide sepsis screening protocols across the United States for more than 20 years (**Box 1**). However, these criteria have been found to be nonspecific to the patient diagnosed with sepsis and less predictive of the septic patient's risk for in-hospital mortality in comparison with organ dysfunction assessments.[2,5] A patient can meet SIRS criteria in nonseptic conditions such as a simple upper respiratory viral infection or in people who have undergone recent vigorous exercise. The sequential organ failure assessment (SOFA) and quick SOFA (qSOFA) scores can be useful for sepsis screening at the time of presentation to the ED (see **Box 1**).[2] The SOFA and qSOFA scores were originally used to assist medical providers' ability to identify intensive care unit patients at high risk for in-hospital mortality. However, the predictive validity of either of the SOFA scores was greater than SIRS criteria.[1,2]

The SOFA score ranges from 0 to 5 and consists of an evaluation of 6 organ systems: respiratory, renal, hepatic, cardiovascular, hematological, and neurologic.

Box 1
Systemic inflammatory response syndrome

Temperature greater than or equal to 38°C or less than 36°F

Heart rate greater than 92

Respiratory rate greater than 20/min or $Paco_2$ less than 32

White blood cell count greater than 1200/mm² or less than 4000/mm² or greater than 10% immature bands

Data from Rhodes A, Alhazzani W, Antonelli M, et al. Surviving sepsis campaign: international guidelines for management of sepsis and septic shock: 2016. Soc Crit Care Med 2017;45(3):1–29.

The qSOFA ranges from 0 to 3 and calculates 1 point for each of the following: (a) increased respiratory rate over 22 per minute; (b) altered mental status measured by abnormal Glasgow Coma Scale less than 15; and (c) a systolic blood pressure less than 100 mm Hg.[5] Patients with scores of 2 or higher have a 3- to 14-fold increase for in-hospital mortality than those with scores less than 2.[2]

In the ED, the qSOFA can be used in triage or before serum laboratories are resulted to promptly identify patients suspicious for sepsis or septic shock.[5] The SOFA scores are not recognized as diagnostic tools but can be useful in emergency settings to help differentiate patients with sepsis when more specific measures are not available. In the ED when patients are undifferentiated but infection is suspected, the predictive validity for mortality using qSOFA was statistically greater than the use of SOFA or SIRS[5] (**Table 1**).

Laboratory Findings

As previously mentioned, evidence of organ dysfunction has more clinical utility in identifying the septic patient than using SIRS criteria alone. Evidence of organ dysfunction is most reliably identified via serum laboratory surveillance and are the data used to calculate the SOFA score (**Table 2**). Routine studies to evaluate patients for sepsis include a complete blood count (CBC), comprehensive metabolic panel (CMP), lactic acid level, coagulation studies, and blood cultures. Cultures from suspected sources (eg, sputum, urine, wound, etc.) should also be obtained and studied. Arterial blood gases can be obtained to evaluate the patient's oxygenation and acid-base status. The only laboratory data specific to sepsis are those identifying the causative organism. Otherwise, laboratory data are used to provide evidence of inflammation, oxygenation and volume status, and organ function.[3]

The CBC can be evaluated for leukocytosis, bandemia, thrombocytopenia, and anemia or hemoconcentration. The CMP can be evaluated for electrolyte imbalances, hyperglycemia, and kidney and/or liver function. A glucose level greater than 140 mg/dL in the absence of diabetes is congruent with increased physiologic stress due to systemic pathologies such as sepsis. Hyperlactatemia with levels greater than 2 mmol/L can be a significant indicator of tissue hypoperfusion even in the absence of hypotension or other signs of shock.[3] Coagulopathies can be identified when the internalized normalized ration is greater than 1.5 or when the activated partial thromboplastin time is greater than 60 seconds.[5,6]

EARLY MANAGEMENT OF THE ADULT SEPTIC PATIENT

In a study published by the New England Journal of Medicine, 49,331 adult patients seen in the ED of 149 hospitals received protocolized sepsis management via a bundle of interventions that were completed in the first 3 hours of care.[4] According to the Surviving Sepsis Campaign, a 36% to 40% reduction of the odds of dying in the hospital

Table 1 Quick sequential organ failure assessment	
Systolic Blood Pressure	Less than or equal to 100 mm/hg
Respiratory Rate	Greater than or equal to 22 breaths/min
Glascow Coma Scale	Less than 15

Data from Seymour CW, Liu VX, Iwashyna TJ, et al. Assessment of clinical criteria for sepsis. JAMA 2016;315(8):762–74.

Table 2
Sequential organ failure assessment

	0	1	2	3	4
Respiratory Pao$_2$:Fio$_2$ ratio (mm Hg)	>400	>400	≤300	≤200[a]	≤100[a]
Renal Creatinine (mg/dL) or actual urine output (mL/d)	<1.2	1.2–1.9	2.0–3.4	3.5–4.9 or <500 Ml/d	≤5 or <200 Ml/d
Hepatic Total bilirubin (mg/dL)	<1.2	1.2–1.9	2.0–5.9	6.0–11.9	12 and >
Cardiovascular Mean arterial pressure (mm Hg)	No evidence of hypotension	MAP <70	Dopamine ≤5 or dobutamine (any dose)	Dopamine >5 or epinephrine ≤0.1	Dopamine >15 or epinephrine >0.1
Hematological Platelet count (×10^3/mm^3)	>150	≤150	≤100	≤50	≤20
Neurologic Glasgow Coma Score	15	13–14	10–12	6–9	<6

[a] With support from mechanical ventilation.
Data from Seymour CW, Liu VX, Iwashyna TJ, et al. Assessment of clinical criteria for sepsis. JAMA 2016;315(8):762–74.

when compliance with either the 3-hour or the 6-hour bundles took place.[1] The 3-hour bundle is preferred in the ED and consists of measuring a lactate level, obtaining blood cultures before the administration of antibiotics, administration of broad spectrum antibiotics, and the administration of a crystalloid fluid at 30 mL/kg of body weight.[1] Early source control with the administration of broad-spectrum antibiotics was found to improve the patient's risk for in-hospital mortality. There was no positive correlation of early fluid resuscitation to in-hospital mortality. It was also determined that the longer time to completion of the 3-hour bundle and delay in administration of antibiotics caused increased risk for in-hospital mortality.[4] During a study conducted from 2009 to 2014, it was determined that admission rates for sepsis has largely remained the same but a decrease in in-hospital mortality only decreased by 3%.[5] This can be interpreted as an indicator that closer attention should be made to earlier detection and treatment.

Antimicrobial Initiation

Gram-negative bacteria are the most common causative organism for sepsis; however, gram-positive bacteria are a virulent organism responsible for sepsis as well. Broad spectrum antibiotics should include therapies able to treat gram-positive and gram-negative organisms. Sepsis resulting from nosocomial infections such as methicillin-resistant *Staphylococcus aureus* (MRSA) has higher patient mortality rates when compared with community-acquired infections.[7] The goal is to begin early, appropriate antimicrobial treatment against the infecting organism.

This diagnosis is made on physical examination, clinical presentation, and clinician's index of suspicion. Radiographic evidence of pneumonia or urinalysis containing bacteria and/or white blood cells can be used to confirm suspicion. The anatomic site of infection is likely to be the most important factor in treatment with respect to the typical pathogen profile and the effectiveness of the antimicrobial to penetrate the site.[1] Another consideration in selecting an antimicrobial therapy is to determine the prevalence of pathogens within the community, for the newly presenting patient, and hospital for those patients who are recently discharged. If the pathogen is known or there is reason to highly suspect a pathogen, the resistance patterns of the pathogen should be considered.[1]

Initial empirical antimicrobial therapy should be broad enough to cover pathogens isolated in health care–associated infections.[1,8] A broad-spectrum carbapenem, such as meropenem, imipenem/cilastatin, or doripenem, is recommended for initial treatment. An extended-range penicillin/β-lactamase inhibitor combination, such as piperacillin/tazobactam or ticarcillin/clavulanate, may also be considered. If a multidrug regimen is required, adding a third- or higher-generation cephalosporin should be considered. In addition to those mentioned earlier, a supplemental gram-negative agent is recommended for critically ill septic patients.[1]

Vancomycin or another anti-MRSA should be used when MRSA is known or suspected, such as with cellulitis. If Legionella is suspected, the addition of a macrolide or fluoroquinolone is most appropriate.[1] If the risk of Candida is suspected to be the cause of sepsis, the selection of the antifungal agent should be adjusted to the severity of the presenting infection.[1]

Fluid Resuscitation

Initial fluid resuscitation in sepsis and septic shock should begin immediately to prevent or correct sepsis-induced hypoperfusion. At least 30 mL/kg of body weight of intravenous crystalloid fluid should be infused within the first 3 hours of presentation to the ED.[1] Failure to aggressively attempt to restore perfusion may contribute to higher mortality rates and treatment failure. Intravascular hypovolemia many be severe in sepsis and requires rapid infusion of large volumes unless there is evidence of pulmonary edema.[1]

The goal of initial fluid resuscitation is to achieve tissue perfusion and stabilize hemodynamic response to systemic infection. Crystalloid infusions such as normal saline or Ringer lactate are largely considered to be therapeutic and most often used in clinical practice.[1]

The use of albumin is appropriate in patients who require several crystalloids to correct the hypoperfusion state, whereas hydroxyethyl starches are not recommended.[1] It is important for the clinician to be judicious with fluid resuscitation in patients at risk for volume overload or cerebral edema.

Shock Management

As previously mentioned, septic shock is redefined as "sepsis with circulatory and cellular/metabolic dysfunction associated with a higher risk of mortality."[1]

Patients presenting to the ED in septic shock are not only undifferentiated from nonseptic etiologic factors but also are at an increased risk for death if not appropriately screened and identified as septic. Shock management for the septic patient is similar to other distributive shocks and is hinged on appropriate volume resuscitation supporting both circulatory and metabolic demands. However, given the high risk for mortality, sepsis research suggests goal-directed resuscitative efforts are most effective against septic shock related mortality.[1]

Circulatory shock is clinically evidenced by a mean arterial pressure less than 60 mm Hg and evidence of poor systemic perfusion. A familiar indicator for poor systemic perfusion is the lactic acid level. For a lactic acid level greater than 4 mmol/L, volume resuscitation with a crystalloid solution should be started with a 30 mL/kg bolus. Circulatory support should be guided by maintaining a mean arterial pressure (MAP) greater than 65 mm Hg or to a normal lactate level. Fluid responsiveness can be determined by central venous pressure monitoring when a central venous catheter is placed. However, the best means to measure fluid responsiveness is with bedside ultrasound, measuring inferior vena cava compressibility. When the patient is no longer fluid responsive or fluid resuscitation does not achieve an MAP greater than 65 mm Hg, norepinephrine is the first-line vasopressor agent recommended for septic shock.[2] When the undifferentiated shock patient presents to the ED, crystalloid fluid resuscitation and/or initiating norepinephrine are optimal choices for early shock management (**Table 3**).

Interprofessional Communication

Improving communication among all clinicians caring for the septic patient also improves the timeliness, efficiency, and overall quality of care. Caregivers initiating therapies in the ED should communicate the patient's presentation, any family or next-of-kin accompanying the patient, diagnostic tests completed, therapies rendered, and the patient's response to therapies to inpatient caregivers.[1] The time antimicrobial agents were initiated is vital to both pharmacy and nursing staff's accuracy of timing subsequent doses. Pertinent test results that may suggest the infectious source communicated to inpatient providers can facilitate evaluation of adequate source control. The patient's response to fluid or vasopressor resuscitation is also a relevant information that is helpful in facilitating continuity of care. Last but not least, ED clinicians should facilitate the integration of the patient's family with the plan of care and ensure the family's wishes are communicated during hand-off reports.[1]

SUMMARY

Sepsis and septic shock are medical emergencies associated with high mortality rates. Early recognition and management of patients with sepsis or septic shock with evidence-based goal-directed medical therapies reduces the patient's risk for death. Implications for future nursing practice include the need for increased vigilance for the clinical indicators associated with sepsis and use of the newly recommended tools (qSOFA or SOFA) for sepsis screening (**Table 4**). As sepsis research continues to evolve, the need for future research should include studying the use of an early consultation system and specific hand-off communication tool for ED and critical care clinicians aimed to facilitate smooth transition of care.

Table 3
Surviving sepsis recommendations and rationales

1. Initial fluid resuscitation	• Begin immediately • Correct hypoperfusion at least 30 mL/kg in first 3 h • Continuous, invasive if necessary, monitoring of hemodynamic status and cardiac function for target mean arterial pressure of 65 mmHg • Resuscitate until lactate normalizes
2. Hospitals have a performance improvement program for sepsis and sepsis screening for all acutely ill patients	• Early recognition using qSOFA • Early treatment using 3 or 6 h bundle
3. Diagnosis	• Blood cultures to be obtained before beginning antibiotic treatment (unless this causes a substantial delay in care) • Two sets of blood cultures are recommended (aerobic and anaerobic)
4. Antimicrobial treatment	• Broad spectrum • One or more antimicrobials are recommended • Narrow antimicrobial treatment after pathogen identified • Consider age and comorbidities (renal and hepatic dosing; immune status) • Avoid sustained empirical antimicrobial use in inflammatory, noninfectious processes (pancreatitis)
5. Source control	• Consider anatomic source of infection • Remove any invasive device thought to be the source (central venous catheter)
6. Fluid Therapy	• Use either balanced crystalloids or saline for fluid resuscitation of patients with sepsis or septic shock • Add albumin when patients require substantial amounts of crystalloids • Avoid using hydroxyethyl starches for intravascular volume replacement • Use crystalloids over gelatins when resuscitating patients
7. Vasoactive medications (central and arterial lines recommended)	• First-line: norepinephrine • Consider adding either vasopressin or norepinephrine to increase mean arterial pressure to target • Dopamine is an alternative agent to norepinephrine only in selected patients • Do not use dopamine for renal protection • Use dobutamine in patients with persistent hypoperfusion despite adequate fluid loading and the use of vasopressor agents
8. Corticosteroids	• Do not use IV hydrocortisone if adequate fluid resuscitation and vasopressor therapy restore hemodynamic stability • If hemodynamic stability cannot be achieved, IV hydrocortisone at a dose of 200 mg/d is recommended
9. Blood products	• Transfuse packed red blood cells only when hemoglobin is <7.0 g/dL • Transfuse prophylactic platelets when <10,000/mm³. • If no bleeding is apparent but patient is at risk for bleeding then transfuse when platelets are <20,000/mm³
10. Immunoglobulins/ blood purification/ antithrombin	• Not recommended in the treatment of sepsis

Abbreviation: IV, intravenous.

Adapted from Rhodes A, Evans L, Alhazzani W. Surviving sepsis campaign: international guidelines for management of sepsis and septic shock: 2016. Crit Care Med 2017;45(3):486–552; with permission.

Table 4
Laboratory study changes in sepsis

Possible Changes Seen with Sepsis	Normal Values
White cell count: • >12,000 uL^{-1} • <4000 uL^{-1}	• 4000–12,000 uL^{-1}
Platelets: • <100 × 10^{-3}/ul	• 150–300 × 10^{-3}/ul
International normalized ratio: • >1.5	• <1.5
Lactate: • >2 mmol/L (hyperlactatemia) • >4 mmol/L (lactic acidosis)	• <2 mmol/L
Partial pressure of oxygen/fraction of inspired oxygen: • <300	• >400

REFERENCES

1. Rhodes A, Alhazzani W, Antonelli M, et al. Surviving sepsis campaign: international guidelines of sepsis and septic shock: 2016. Soc Crit Care Med 2017;45(3):1–29.
2. Singer M, Deutschman CS, Seymour CW. The third international consensus definitions for sepsis and septic shock (Sepsis-3). JAMA 2016;315(8):801–10.
3. Sweet D, Marsden J, Kendall H, et al. Emergency management of sepsis: the simple stuff saves lives. B C Med J 2012;54(4):176–82.
4. Seymour CW, Gesten F, Prescott HC. Time to treatment and mortality during mandated emergency care for sepsis. N Engl J Med 2017;376(23):2235–44.
5. Seymour CW, Liu VX, Iwashyna TJ, et al. Assessment of clinical criteria for sepsis. J Am Med Assoc 2016;315(8):762–74.
6. Adams JG. Emergency medicine clinical essentials. 2nd edition. Philadelphia: Elsevier; 2013.
7. Labelle A, Juang P, Reichley R, et al. The determinants of hospital mortality among patients with septic shock receiving appropriate antibiotic therapy. J Crit Care Med 2012;40:2016.
8. Martin GS, Mannino DM, Easton S, et al. The epidemiology of sepsis in the United States from 1979 through 2000. N Engl J Med 2003;348:1546.

Sepsis in the Obstetric Client

Marie Adorno, PhD, APRN, CNS, RNC

KEYWORDS

- Maternal sepsis • Puerperal infections • PROM • Mastitis • Endometritis
- Urinary tract infections

KEY POINTS

- When caring for obstetric patients, it is important to identify the stages of prenatal (antepartum), labor and delivery (intrapartum), and postpartum care.
- During the initial weeks of pregnancy, bodily changes can ultimately affect the health of both the mother and the newborn.
- Identification of the signs and symptoms associated with sepsis in obstetric patients may be difficult, as pregnant patients goes through bodily changes.
- Most postpartum infections take place after hospital discharge and in the absence of postnatal follow-up. Consequently, some cases of puerperal infections remain undiagnosed and unreported.

According to the World Health Organization (WHO), maternal sepsis is "a life-threatening condition defined as organ dysfunction resulting from infection during pregnancy, childbirth, post-abortion, or postpartum period."[1] Maternal sepsis is the third most common direct cause of maternal mortality following maternal hemorrhage and maternal hypertension.[2] Undetected and poorly managed maternal infections lead to sepsis, death, or disability for the mother and an increased likelihood of early neonatal infection and other adverse outcomes. When caring for obstetric patients, it is important to identify the stages of obstetric care: prenatal (antepartum), labor and delivery (intrapartum), and after the birth of the infant (postpartum). Sepsis occurs at any stage of obstetric care. Assessment and identification of risk factors assist with recognizing potential problems. Health care providers must remain mindful of the bodily changes that occur during the initial weeks of pregnancy, while assessing for potential problems that could ultimately affect the health of both the mother and the newborn during delivery and in the postpartum period.[1,2]

Several organizations and researchers have recognized the need to address the causes of maternal and newborn mortality and morbidity. Bonet and colleagues[3] (2018) conducted the Global Maternal Sepsis Study (GLOSS). The purpose of the

Disclosure: The author has nothing to disclose.
Department of Nursing, LSU Health New Orleans School of Nursing, 1900 Gravier Street, New Orleans, LA 70112, USA
E-mail address: madorn@lsuhsc.edu

study was to establish criteria for the identification of possible severe maternal infection and maternal sepsis. The GLOSS also reinforced the importance of building a network of health care facilities to implement quality improvement strategies for better identification and management of maternal and early neonatal sepsis.

MATERNAL SEPSIS

Maternal sepsis is reported as the underlying cause for 11% of all maternal deaths.[3] Maternal infections are common because of the physiologic changes of pregnancy. Sepsis is characterized by a systematic response to an invasive organism. The changes that occur in the maternal immune responses during pregnancy predispose the pregnant patient to develop infections that would not otherwise cause a problem in the nonpregnant state. Identification of the signs and symptoms associated with sepsis in obstetric patients may be harder, as the pregnant woman goes through bodily changes that may mask the signs of sepsis. Clinical signs and symptoms of sepsis are changes in body temperature including hypothermia and hyperthermia, tachycardia (heart rate >110), and either high or low white blood cell count (WBC). WBC as an indicator for infection is difficult, as the WBC may be elevated during pregnancy and especially at birth and an increase in body temperature is commonly seen during labor.[2]

Antepartum

There are several antepartum infections that clinicians must assess for during the antepartum stage of pregnancy. These infections include urinary tract infections (UTIs), cystitis, vaginal infections, respiratory infections, and group B streptococcus (GBS) disease.

INFECTIONS

UTIs are common during pregnancy because of physiologic changes in the urinary tract that contribute to urinary stasis. Cystitis is inflammation of the bladder caused by UTIs. Cystitis can lead to pyelonephritis with symptoms of dysuria, a high fever, retropubic or suprapubic pain, flank pain, or tenderness. Exogenous bacteria introduced from an external source, such as contaminated gloves or instruments, droplet infections, or foreign objects inserted into the vagina, can cause vaginal infections. Sexually transmitted diseases may cause uterine infections if left untreated during pregnancy.[4]

Acute or chronic respiratory tract infections also may occur during pregnancy as a result of the physiologic changes that occur in the respiratory system. Acute conditions include bronchitis, pneumonia, and pleurisy; chronic conditions include pulmonary tuberculosis and chronic bronchitis.[4]

GROUP B STREPTOCOCCUS

GBS is a perinatal pathogen that causes infection in the antepartum period that can contribute to neonatal and maternal complications.[5] In the 1970s, GBS emerged as the leading infectious cause of early neonatal morbidity and mortality in the United States and remains the leading infectious disease of mortality and morbidity of newborns in the United States. The primary risk factor for GBS is maternal colonization with GBS in the genitourinary or gastrointestinal tracts. GBS is a gram-positive bacterium that causes invasive disease primarily in infants, pregnant or postpartum women, and older adults, with the highest incidence among young infants. Infections in newborns occurring within the first week of life are designated early onset disease.

Late-onset infections occur in infants aged greater than 1 week, with most infections evident during the first 3 months of life.[6]

Recommendations for intrapartum antibiotic prophylaxis to prevent perinatal GBS disease were issued in 1996 by the American College of Obstetricians and Gynecologists and the Centers for Disease Control and Prevention and in 1997 by the American Academy of Pediatrics. Revised guidelines for the prevention of early onset GBS disease issued in 2002 recommended universal culture-based screening of all pregnant women at 35 to 37 weeks' gestation to optimize the identification of women who should receive intrapartum antibiotic prophylaxis and to prepare for potential complications in the delivery period. Medical treatment of decreasing potential side effects of positive GBS includes administering intravenous antibiotics at the onset of labor and every 4 hours until delivery of infant.[6]

Although the guidelines focus on interventions to prevent early onset GBS disease, the same measures may prevent some perinatal maternal infections. Infants with early onset GBS disease generally present with respiratory distress, apnea, or other signs of sepsis within the first 24 to 48 hours of life. The most common clinical problems are sepsis and pneumonia with some early-onset infections leading to meningitis.[6]

Maternal intrapartum GBS colonization is the primary risk factor for early onset disease in infants. In addition to maternal colonization with GBS, other factors that increase the risk for early-onset disease include gestational age less than 37 completed weeks, membrane rupture of greater than 12 hours, temperature greater than 99.5°F (>37.5°C), intra-amniotic infection, young maternal age, black race, and low maternal levels of GBS-specific anticapsular antibody. Previous delivery of an infant with invasive GBS disease is a risk factor for early onset disease in future deliveries.[6]

Intrapartum

Several infections may occur during the intrapartum (labor and delivery) period, including intra-amniotic infection, premature rupture of membranes, and maternal bacteremia. Ongoing assessment of signs and symptoms will assist the health care provider to initiate interventions that will benefit both the mother and the newborn and prevent complications of infection or sepsis.

INTRA-AMNIOTIC INFECTION

"Intra-amniotic infection (IAI), formerly called chorioamnionitis, is a complication of pregnancy caused by bacterial infection of the fetal amnionic and chorionic membranes."[7] The IAI is most often associated with prolonged labor and can result in labor abnormalities and the need for cesarean delivery as well as an increased risk of postpartum hemorrhage. Diagnostic criteria for IAI include maternal fever greater than 100.4°F (>38°C) and at least 2 of the following clinical findings: uterine tenderness, maternal tachycardia (>100 beats per minute [bpm]), fetal tachycardia (>160 bpm), maternal leukocytosis (15,000 WBC/mm^3), and/or purulent or foul-smelling amniotic fluid.[6] Assessment and early identification are necessary to assist the mother, fetus, and neonate. The activation of maternal and fetal inflammatory responses may result in the clinical signs and symptoms of sepsis in the neonate. The maternal response is manifested by inflammation of the chorioamnion, and the fetal response is manifested by inflammation of the umbilical cord.[7]

Neonates have an immature immune system and are unable to stimulate a bone marrow response. The reserve of neutrophils is easily depleted and, therefore, unable to destroy the bacteria. The replication of bacteria results in systemic illness in the neonate. The initial attempt of the neonate immune system to respond to the inflammatory process has a physiologic impact on the neonate's organ systems with the result of early onset sepsis (EOS).[7]

When anticipating a birth with possible IAI, the nurse should focus care based on the following assessment criteria to assist with identifying the possibility of EOS in the newborn[7]:

- Maternal temperature of greater than 100.4°F (>38°C)
- Maternal and/or fetal tachycardia
- Ruptured membranes for greater than 18 hours
- Foul-smelling amniotic fluid present
- Maternal-positive GBS status

The clinical diagnosis of sepsis at birth is difficult because the signs and symptoms are nonspecific. Ongoing assessment and documentation to monitor the infant's condition for subtle changes over the first days of life are important. Sepsis occurring in the neonate secondary to IAI usually appears within the first 24 hours of life. Therefore, it is important to recognize early signs and symptoms of neonatal sepsis.[7]

PREMATURE RUPTURE OF MEMBRANES

Premature rupture of membranes (PROM) occurs in 5% to 10% of all pregnancies. Approximately 60% of cases are term pregnancies and are associated with complications of maternal and neonatal infections. Dundar and colleagues[8] (2018) conducted a retrospective case-control study that related complications of maternal and neonatal infections with preterm PROM (PPROM). PPROM occurs before 37 weeks of gestation. Dundar and colleagues[8] concluded that the expected management is antibiotic prophylaxis prescribed for a maximum of 10 days or until labor starts spontaneously. Labor was induced if infection was suspected; the newborns who were part of the study met the following neonatal intensive care unit admission criteria: transient problems requiring cardiorespiratory monitoring, need for peripheral intravenous fluid therapy, jaundiced infants requiring peripheral intravenous fluid therapy and closer monitoring, preterm at less than 32 weeks of gestation, respiratory distress syndrome (RDS), neonatal sepsis, exchange transfusion, and sustained assisted ventilation.

In the study conducted by Dundar and colleagues,[8] a diagnosis of sepsis was made with the presence of at least 3 of the following: temperature instability, tachypnea (>70/min), feeding intolerance, abdominal distension, hepatosplenomegaly, dyspnea, lethargy, tachycardia (heart rate >190 bpm), and bradycardia (heart rate <90 bpm). Infants with respiratory distress, tachypnea, nasal flaring, grunting and a grainy shadow, and air bronchogram and a white lung in the chest radiograph were diagnosed with RDS.

Dundar and colleagues[8] concluded that the most common and serious complications of PPROM are RDS, intraventricular hemorrhage, necrotizing enterocolitis, and sepsis. As the time interval between membrane rupture and delivery increases, the risk of maternal and neonatal infections also increases. Problems can also surface in the postpartum period either independently of issues that occurred or with problems from the prenatal period, such as UTIs.

NEWBORN SEPSIS

"Newborn sepsis remains one of the top 10 leading causes of death in neonates in the United States. Seventy-five percent of all neonatal deaths worldwide occur during the first week of life, and 25% to 44% occur within the first 24 hours of life."[1] Early identification of clinical signs and symptoms of infection could improve outcomes and prevent neonatal deaths. Diagnosis of sepsis can be difficult because there are many subtle signs and symptoms and there are no standard guidelines that define clinical manifestations. Neonatal sepsis is defined as a bacterial infection in the blood, which is classified by day of life at diagnosis. EOS develops within the first 2 to 3 days after birth, and late-onset sepsis occurs within 3 to 7 days or as late as 120 days after birth.[1,9]

PERIPARTUM MATERNAL BACTEREMIA

Maternal sepsis is an important contributor to severe maternal morbidity. Peripartum maternal bacteremia is an infection that occurs during pregnancy or in the intrapartum period, which is the time of labor and delivery of the infant. Guidelines for encouraging early diagnosis and treatment of febrile women during labor and delivery conflict with evidence-based recommendations. Additionally, there is no current gold standard for the diagnosis of sepsis in pregnancy.[10]

Easter and colleagues[10] (2017) conducted a case-control study that evaluated the degree of initial fever as a clinical predictor. The tertiary care centers where the study was conducted used a guideline-based maternal fever protocol, including the collection of 2 sets of blood cultures, laboratory studies, and initiation of antibiotics (ampicillin or penicillin) for all pregnant and postpartum women with a single fever of 100.4°F or greater. The results showed that maternal bacteremia is associated with an initial fever greater than 100.4°F during labor and a fever of 102°F or greater.[10] Therefore, clinical manifestations in the intrapartum period must be reported to the health care providers caring for patients in the postpartum period so that early intervention can assist with decreasing risk factors associated with infection.

Postpartum

The postpartum period begins immediately after the birth of an infant and extends to approximately 6 weeks as the maternal hormones and uterine size return to a nonpregnant state. The WHO reports that most maternal and newborn deaths occur during the postpartum period.[1]

PUERPERAL INFECTION

Puerperal infection is the major cause of maternal morbidity and mortality in the United States and occurs in the postpartum period after birth of the infant. Puerperal infection is defined as a bacterial infection of the genital tract that occurs within 28 days after miscarriage, induced abortion, or childbirth. Infections during the postpartum period occur in the endometrium (endometritis); operative wound site, such as a cesarean incision or episiotomy; urinary tract, and breasts (mastitis).[1,4,11]

Puerperal infection is diagnosed with a temperature of 100.4°F or greater ($\geq$38°C) on 2 consecutive days of the first 10 postpartum days and is measured orally at least 4 hours apart. However, the nurse should be aware that postpartum patients may have an elevated temperature in the first 24 hours after delivery due to the body's physiologic response to the stress of delivery.[11]

Mothers who give birth by cesarean delivery have a greater incidence of puerperal infection than mothers who give birth vaginally. Prolonged labor followed by a cesarean delivery increases the incidence of postpartum infection to 30% to 35%.[11] It is important to note that puerperal infections often occur after patients are discharged from the hospital; therefore, nurses must educate patients and family members to the signs and symptoms that must be reported to the health care provider.[11]

ENDOMETRITIS

During the immediate postpartum period, the most common site of infection is the uterine endometrium. The clinical manifestation of endometritis is a temperature elevation greater than 101°F (>38.4°C) occurring within the first 24 to 48 hours after childbirth, followed by uterine tenderness and foul-smelling lochia. Because UTIs could occur during any part of the pregnancy and in the postpartum period, differentiating the signs and symptoms of endometritis and UTI are important.[11]

MASTITIS

Mastitis or breast abscess is a late-appearing infection in the breast tissue, usually unilateral, and develops after the flow of milk has been established. Mastitis is most commonly caused by *Staphylococcus aureus*, which is introduced from the infant's mouth through a crack in the nipple. The infection involves the ductal system, causing inflammatory edema, enlarged axillary lymph nodes, and breast engorgement with obstruction of milk flow.[11]

Symptoms of mastitis are fever, malaise, and localized breast tenderness. Primary management for mastitis includes antibiotic therapy, application of heat or cold to the breasts, hydration, and analgesics. To maintain lactation, the woman is encouraged to breastfeed every 2 to 4 hours or empty the breasts by manual expression or breast pump. Mastitis usually occurs after patients are discharged from the hospital; therefore, an important component of nursing care includes teaching the breastfeeding mother about signs of mastitis and strategies to prevent cracked nipples.[11]

Accurate nursing assessment in recognizing clinical indicators of sepsis is important for the delivery of safe, effective nursing care in the postpartum period. The patients' mental status, vital signs, breasts, fundus, lochia, incisions, and urinary status must be monitored. Temperature elevation may be the first indication of an infection. The nurse must notify the primary care provider immediately if an elevated temperature presents with tachycardia, uterine or fundal tenderness or pain, foul-smelling lochia, an absence or decrease in lochia, chills, decreased appetite, malaise, elevated WBC, back pain, generalized aching, headache, dysuria, urinary frequency or retention, wound drainage, erythema, or edema. Complete blood count with differential, urinalysis with culture and sensitivity, cervical, uterine, or wound cultures should be collected to identify sources of puerperal infections. Blood cultures should be collected if sepsis is suspected.[11]

Prompt treatment is initiated after assessment and diagnosis of maternal infection or sepsis. All bacterial puerperal infections require treatment with antibiotics. The nurse must encourage rest and increased fluid intake and reinforce the importance of increasing protein and vitamin C in the diet. Nurses should refer patients to a

Table 1			
Causes of sepsis during antepartum, intrapartum, and postpartum phases of obstetric care			
Prenatal (Antepartum)	Labor and Delivery (Intrapartum)	Postpartum	Newborn
GBS	Episiotomy	Mastitis	GBS
PROM • Necrotizing enterocolitis • Sepsis	Lacerations	Puerperal infections • Mastitis • Bacteremia	Meningitis
UTIs	—	—	—

Table 2
Clinical signs and symptoms to identify maternal and newborn infections

Prenatal	Labor and Delivery	Postpartum	Newborn
Temp >100.4°F	Temp >100.4°F	Temp >100.4°F	Temp may not be reliable indicator
Tachycardia >100	Maternal tachycardia >100 FHT >120	Tachycardia >100	Tachycardia >120
Changes in sensorium	Changes in sensorium	Changes in sensorium	Subtle behavior changes
UTI Painful urination	—	Boggy uterus UTI Painful urination	—

Abbreviations: FHT, fetal heart tone; temp, temperature.

dietitian when needed. Comfort measures are also important in facilitating patients' full recovery. Cool showers, sitz baths, warm compresses applied to the breasts, therapeutic touch and massage, soothing music, relaxation techniques, pain medications, and antipyretics promote optimal patient care. Nonsteroidal antiinflammatory medications are also used in the treatment plan because of the antiinflammatory effect.[11] Throughout the course of treatment, health care team members must provide education to patients and family members regarding the patients' diagnosis and prognosis, treatment plan, measures to promote good hygiene, and follow-up care[11] **(Table 1)**.

SUMMARY

Maternal sepsis remains a significant contributor to maternal morbidity. The incidence of obstetric-related sepsis in the United States has decreased, yet the consequences of morbidity and mortality are great for those patients with infections. Caregivers and health care providers are required to evaluate newborns and infants for sepsis.[9] When caring for obstetric patients, it is important to recognize that infections or sepsis occur at all stages of obstetric care: prenatal (antepartum), labor and delivery (intrapartum), and after the birth of the infant (postpartum care). Health care providers must remain diligent in assessing risk factors and recognizing potential problems that could lead to sepsis for both the mother and the newborn **(Table 2)**.

REFERENCES

1. World Health Organization (WHO). Statement on maternal sepsis. 2017. Available at: https://www.world-sepsis-day.org/news/2018/1/9/who-statement-on-maternal-sepsis. Accessed February 20, 2018.
2. Parfitt SE, Bogat ML, Hering SH, et al. Sepsis in obstetrics. Clinical features and early warning tools. MCN Am J Matern Child Nurs 2017;42(4):199–205.
3. Bonet M, Souza JP, Edgardo A, et al. The global maternal sepsis study and awareness campaign (GLOSS): study protocol. Reprod Health 2018;15:16.
4. Burke C. Perinatal sepsis. J Perinat Neonatal Nurs 2009;23:42–51.
5. Seale AC, Bianchi-Jassir F, Russel NL, et al. Estimates of the burden of group B streptococcal disease worldwide for pregnant women, stillbirths, and children. Clin Infect Dis 2017;65(S2):S200–19.

6. CDC. Prevention of perinatal group B streptococcal disease: revised guidelines from CDC. Recommendations and Reports 2010;59(RR10):1–322010. Available at: https://www.cdc.gov/mmwr/preview/mmwrhtml/rr5910a1.htm. Accessed February 20, 2018.
7. Raines DA, Wagner A, Salinas A. Intraamniotic infection and the term neonate. Neonatal Netw 2017;36:385–7.
8. Dundar B, Cakmak BD, Ozgen G, et al. Platelet indices in preterm premature rupture of membranes and their relation with adverse neonatal outcomes. J Obstet Gynaecol Res 2018;44(1):67–73.
9. Boettiger M, Tyler-Viola L, Hagan J. Nurses' early recognition of neonatal sepsis. J Obstet Gynecol Neonatal Nurs 2017;46:834–45.
10. Easter SR, Molina RL, Venkatesh KK, et al. Clinical risk factors associated with peripartum maternal bacteremia. Obstet Gynecol 2017;120:710–7.
11. Ward SL, Hisley SM. Maternal-child nursing: optimizing outcomes for mothers, children and families across care settings. 2nd edition. Philadelphia: F.A. Davis; 2015.

Sepsis in the Burn Patient

Check for updates

Jennifer Manning, DNS, APRN, ACNS-BC, CNE

KEYWORDS

• Sepsis • Infection • Burn • Burn treatment • Infection prevention

KEY POINTS

- Sepsis is the leading cause of death in burn patients, resulting in up to 50% to 60% of burn injury deaths.
- Because of the destruction of the skin's natural barrier to infection, all burn types are a risk for complications; therefore, all treatments should involve prevention and treatment of infection in the burn patient.
- Clinical presentation of sepsis is similar to clinical presentation of the burn patient without infection, which presents a challenge in differentially diagnosing sepsis in the burn patient.
- Because of the persistent hypermetabolic response, patients will have persistent tachycardia, tachypnea, and/or leukocytosis, and their normal temperature is reset to an average of 38°C.
- Important steps in monitoring the burn patient for infection and subsequent sepsis are continuous monitoring for signs of infection and implementation of preventative measures to prevent infection.

INTRODUCTION

A burn is damage to the skin and loss of the primary barrier to infection.[1] Burned skin is at risk for infection as long as the barrier is absent. If untreated, an infection from a serious burn can be life-threatening and lead to sepsis. Burns can be caused by a range of sources, including thermal (scalding, flame, contact with hot surfaces), electrical, chemical (acids, gasoline, household cleaners, garden products), and radiation. A burn injury can range from minor to severe.[1]

Sepsis is a life-threatening organ dysfunction caused by dysregulated host response to infection; early treatment is critical.[2] Sepsis is the leading cause of death, resulting in up to 50% to 60% of burn injury deaths. Improvements in care outcomes for burn sepsis patients have been slow owing to the common exclusion of burn patients from sepsis research.[2]

The Surviving Sepsis campaign, a campaign that aims to reduce mortality from sepsis, focuses on patients presenting to hospitals with recent signs of infection.[3] Although many patients are affected by burn sepsis, interventions to treat sepsis in

Disclosure: The author has nothing to disclose.
Louisiana State University Health Sciences Center, School of Nursing, 1900 Gravier, New Orleans, LA 70003, USA
E-mail address: jmanni@lsuhsc.edu

burn patients is challenging owing to a lack of specific guidelines. One critical element is differentiating burn sepsis from sepsis to ensure optimal patient treatment.[3]

INCIDENCE AND PREVALENCE

According to the Centers for Disease Control and Prevention (2018), more than 1.5 million people are diagnosed with sepsis each year in the United States.[2] Of this number, 11% of patients developed sepsis from a skin infection. Because of the infection challenges in burn patients, survival from sepsis is especially challenging. As a result, sepsis is the cause of 50–60% of all deaths in patients with severe burns.[4]

The American Burn Association (ABA) reports more than 450,000 patients are treated in emergency rooms for burns annually.[1] Mortality for patients with more than a 40% total body surface area (TBSA) burn is 95%.[5] Approximately 3400 burn patients will not survive their injuries.[1]

Burns and fires are the third leading cause of death in the home, with a fire-related death occurring every 169 minutes.[1] Most admissions to burn centers result from fire or flame burns (44%), followed by scalding injuries caused by wet or moist heat (33%).[1] The widespread impact burns have on health care warrants the understanding of patient assessment and implementation of the most effective treatments based on the most current evidence.[2]

BURN TYPES

Intact skin is vital to preserving several important body functions, including fluid homeostasis, thermoregulation, and protection from infection. The skin plays an important role in essential immunologic and neurosensory body functions, as well as metabolism of important vitamins such as vitamin D.[3] Whenever there is a break in the skin, these body functions are affected. The relationship of burn types with associated physiologic responses and symptoms as they relate to sepsis are described in **Table 1**. Understanding the physiologic responses and symptoms of burn types is appropriate before addressing the unique sepsis issues associated with burn patients.[2]

All burn types, even when minor, are risks for complications if not treated properly. This is due to the destruction of the skin's natural barrier to infection. All treatments should involve prevention and treatment of infection.[3]

RISK FACTORS

Sepsis can develop in any burn patient with an infection. Risk factors include age, preexisting conditions, type of burn, and response to treatment. Patients with the highest risk are the very young and older adults. Patients with additional risk factors include those with a weakened immune system; a chronic illness, such as diabetes, kidney, or liver disease; AIDS, and/or cancer.[6]

Burn patients are more vulnerable to developing sepsis owing to the increased opportunity for infections to become complicated following invasive hospital procures (eg, central line placement). Rising antibiotic resistance is another factor because it results in microbes becoming immune to drugs that would otherwise control infection.[7]

Open burn wounds pose risks for infection and, ultimately, sepsis. The occurrence of sepsis in burn patients is caused by depression in the immune response and a massive systemic inflammatory response (SIRS). Infections commonly resulting from urinary catheters or mechanical ventilation can be complication risks for the burn patient. Treatment of an infection can be further complicated by the increasing prevalence of drug-resistant pathogens worldwide.[4]

Table 1			
Differentiation of burn types with associated physiologic responses and symptoms			
Type of Burn	**Brief Definition**	**Physiologic Responses**	**Symptoms**
First-Degree	Red, no blistered skin	• Most common • Minor burn • Affects only the outer layer of skin (epidermis)	• Pain • Redness • Swelling • Sunburn
Second-Degree	Blisters and some thickening of the skin affected	• Deeper than first-degree • Affects epidermis and dermis (second layer of skin) • If burn is <2 inches, it is considered minor • A burn larger than 2 inches is considered major • A burn is considered major if it affects the face, hands, feet, a major joint, groin, genitals, and/or buttocks	• Pain, redness, swelling • Possible blisters • Breaks in skin • Chance of infection increases
Third-Degree	Widespread thickness with white, leathery appearance	• Serious burns, even if small • Potentially life-threatening • Go through epidermis, dermis, and fat layer	• May not be painful because nerves destroyed, may be pain around the area where burn not as deep • High risk for dehydration, infection, and sepsis • Facial burns, regardless of degree, can affect airway • Burns on lips and/or mouth, coughing, difficult breathing, voice changes, wheezing
Fourth-Degree	All symptoms of a third-degree burn and also extends beyond the skin into bones and tendons	• Serious burns, even if small • Potentially life-threatening • Go through epidermis, dermis, and fat layer into underlying muscle and bone	• Stiff • Charred • Dry • Initial pain not as severe as third-degree burn due to shock and damage to nerve endings • High risk for dehydration, infection and sepsis

Data from Sepsis Alliance. Sepsis and burns—faces of sepsis 2017. Available at: https://www.sepsis.org/sepsis-and/sepsis-and-burns. Accessed January 6, 2018.

Risk factors include any severe burn that results in an open wound and presence of invasive lines, such as urinary catheters, ventilators, central lines, and intravenous lines. Patients who present with or develop fever, increased respiratory rate, increased heart rate, decreased urinary output, decreased organ function, or change in mental status are at risk for further development of infection or worsening infection and, subsequently, sepsis.[6]

UNIQUE CLINICAL PRESENTATION ISSUES FOR BURN PATIENTS WITH SEPSIS

Burns of more than 15% to 20% of TBSA will have a persistent SIRS for months after the burn wound is closed.[8] Owing to persistent hypermetabolic response, patients will have persistent tachycardia, tachypnea, and/or leukocytosis, and their normal temperature is reset to an average of 38°C. This response is due to increased glucose, protein, and lipid metabolism following the onset of the burn (**Fig. 1**). All of these clinical presentations are similar to sepsis signs and present a challenge in differentially diagnosing sepsis in the burn patient. Moreover, this type of presentation requires rapid diagnosis and prompt initiation of treatment. Onset of sepsis is rare in first week following a burn. The risk exists weeks to months following the burn. As long as the burn wound is open, the risk of sepsis exists. With severe burns, patients may experience sepsis multiple times during recovery.[9] Owing to these unique issues, the traditional sepsis bundle may not apply to the burn patient.

Clinical presentation of sepsis results from a temperature greater than 101°F or less than 95°F, a respiratory rate more than 20 breaths per minute, and a heart rate more than 90 beats per minute, as well as pain, redness, and swelling to the infected area. Clinical presentation of septic shock results from a marked decrease in blood pressure, organ failure, difficulty breathing, abnormal heart function, abdominal pain, confusion, and/or disorientation.[10]

DIAGNOSIS

Although patients with large burns often meet the criteria for sepsis, clearer definitions are needed for what should trigger concern for infection in this patient population. According to the ABA, diagnostic criteria for sepsis include progressive tachycardia, progressive tachypnea, thrombocytopenia, hyperglycemia (without preexisting diabetes mellitus), and inability to continue enteral feedings for more than 24 hours.[11] Once these criteria are met, the search for the pathologic source of the infection should ensue.

Important steps include monitoring the burn patient for signs of infection and subsequent sepsis, and implementation of measures to prevent infection. **Table 2** lists the early and late signs of infection in the burn patient.

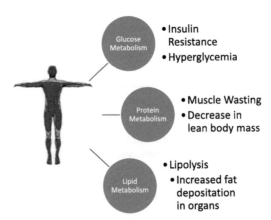

Fig. 1. Metabolism changes based on the hypermetabolic response in the burn patient. (*Adapted from* Bakhtyar N, Sivayoganathan T, Jeschke M. Therapeutic approaches to combatting hypermetabolism in severe burn injuries. J Intens and Crit Care 2015;1:1–12. Available at: http://criticalcare.imedpub.com/therapeutic-approaches-to-combatting-hypermetabolism-insevere-burn-injuries.php?aid=7762.)

Table 2
Early and late signs of infection in burn patients

Early Signs	Late Signs
Fever or hypothermia	Lactic acidosis
Chills	Oliguria
Tachycardia	Leukopenia
Tachypnea	Disseminated intravascular coagulation (DIC)
Nausea, vomiting	Myocardial depression
Hyperglycemia	Pulmonary edema
Lethargy, malaise	Hypotension
Proteinuria	Hypoglycemia
Hypoxia	Azotemia
Leukocytosis	Thrombocytopenia
Hyperbilirubinemia	Acute respiratory distress syndrome (ARDS)
	Gastrointestinal hemorrhage
	Coma

Data from Lavrentieva A, Papadopoulou S, Kioumis J, et al. PCT as a diagnostic and prognostic tool in burn patients. Whether time course has a role in monitoring sepsis treatment. Burns 2012;38:356.

Most microorganisms isolated in burn units are gram-negative pathogens. Gram-negative bacteria have a higher probability of developing resistance to antimicrobials compared with gram-positive bacteria. The most common gram-negative bacteria identified in burn units are *Pseudomonas aeruginosa* (74%), *Escherichia coli* (35%), *Acinetobacter baumannii* (24%), coagulase-negative staphylococci (21%), and *Enterococcus* (14%).[4]

TREATMENT AND MANAGEMENT

There have been many advances in treating sepsis but few advances in treating burn patients with sepsis.[12] In fact, the trigger to initiate care may not always be clear owing to similar presenting symptoms between the burn patient without

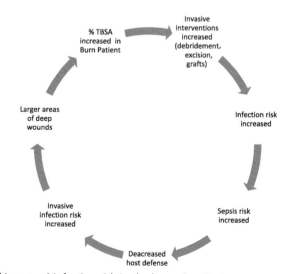

Fig. 2. Cycle of increased infection risk in the burned patient.

infection and the burn patient with infection and/or sepsis.[13] Guidelines regarding antibiotic treatment duration, use of steroids, and optimal hemodynamic support is not always clear for these patients. Sepsis guidelines specific to the burn patient are needed to guide best practices and ultimately improve patient outcomes.[9] The approach to treatment should consider the ongoing cycle of infection risk in burn patients (**Fig. 2**).

Initial patient assessment should include a determination of the burn area, size, and degree. Careful attention should be paid to the face, hands, feet, major joints, groin, genitals, and buttocks; and any burn greater than 2 inches should be assessed. Planning and goal identification should include short-term and long-term recovery for the patient. Short-term goals include stabilizing the patient while preventing infection. Long-term goals include strategies that aim to return the patient to baseline (**Fig. 3**).

Although there are no national sepsis guidelines specific for burn patients, sepsis interventions, including burn care, pharmacologic treatment, monitoring, hypermetabolic response treatment, and prevention measures, should be provided to prevent and treat infection.[13] **Table 3** lists these interventions.

The primary cause of death if the patient survives the initial burn shock resuscitation is septic shock, followed by multiple organ dysfunction syndrome, both results of sepsis.

Outcome evaluation should include short-term and long-term goals. Short-term goals should include preventing worsening of illness, impaired function, frailty, onset of new comorbidity, and immune abnormalities. Long-term goals should include rehabilitation, activities of daily life, coping, and preventing mortality.

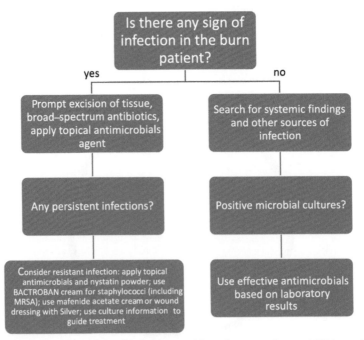

Fig. 3. Management algorithm of infection problems in severe burns. MRSA, methicillin-resistant *Staphylococcus aureus*.

Table 3
Interventions for burn patients with infection

Burn Care	• Do not soak the affected area in water, place ice, or apply ointments • Carefully remove clothing or fabric stuck to burn • For chemical burns, rinse area with water to flush chemical away • Cover affected area with loose sterile cloth or bandage • Administer burn creams as applicable • For nonserious burns, soak in water for a few minutes, then dry (pat), apply aloe vera to relive pain, cover with loose covering only, monitor for infection, do not break blisters • Routine debridement, including blisters covering large surface areas Negative pressure wound dressings, such as wound vacuum-assisted closure (VAC) systems, allow the additions of solutions with application of negative pressure Silver can be used to kill broad-spectrum microorganisms with silver-impregnated dressings or creams • Wound cleansing can include irrigation, swabbing, showering, bathing, washing, or whirlpool baths Saline, water or antiseptic solutions can be used These therapies have had a positive impact on reducing death rates among patients (up to 50%)
Pharmacologic Treatments	• Administer intravenous fluids for hydration • Administer medications for pain • Administer antibiotics for infection • Administer antimicrobial therapy ointments topically
Monitoring	• Seek medical attention for development of any discharge, increased pain, change in color, and/or fever
Sepsis Interventions	• Stabilize heart function, breathing, and blood pressure • Vasopressors can be used to constrict blood vessels and increase blood pressure • Provide oxygen and intravenous fluids Broad-spectrum antibiotics should be quickly administered and switched (as needed) to a more specific antibiotic based on blood tests identifying the source of the infection • Insulin may be used to stabilize blood sugar levels • Corticosteroids may be used • Immune system medications can be administered • Pain relief and sedatives may be provided to treat pain and anxiety
Hypermetabolic Response Treatment	• Early wound excision and closure • Nutrition • Thermoregulation • Exercise • Insulin • Recombinant human growth hormone • Metformin • Propranolol • Oxandrolone
Preventative Measures	• Risk factor for antibiotic-resistant organisms include antibiotics administered before infection development or extended hospitalization • Routine tracking of infection is needed • Short-term antibiotic administration and use of antibiotics based on monitoring of antibiotic resistance trends within burn centers • Prophylactic antibiotics should not be routinely used in burn victim management

Data from Yusuf K. Infection control in severely burned patients. World J Crit Care Med 2012;1(4): 94–101.

SUMMARY

Sepsis in a burn patient is different from sepsis in an unburned patient. Survival from sepsis has not changed dramatically over the past few decades. Efforts have been made to improve the speed of diagnosis and shorten the time for sepsis treatment. This is a challenge because the burn patient has lost the primary barrier to infection, their skin. Another unique complication is the hypermetabolic response that persists for several months in burn patients. Close monitoring is required as long as the burn wound is open. Efforts are needed to develop more accurate diagnostic strategies and guidelines to trigger rapid treatment via sepsis bundles that specifically meet burn patient needs.

REFERENCES

1. American Burn Association (ABA). Burn statistics. 2018. Available at: http://burninjuryguide.com/burn-statistics/.
2. Sepsis. Centers for Disease Control (CDC) and Prevention. 2018. Available at: https://www.cdc.gov/sepsis/datareports/index.html.
3. Sepsis and burns 2017 Sepsis alliance. Available at: https://www.sepsis.org/sepsis-and/sepsis-and-burns/.
4. Wardhana A, Djan R, Halim Z. Bacterial and antimicrobial susceptibility profile and the prevalence of sepsis among burn patients at the burn unit of Cipto Mangunkusumo Hospital. Ann Burns fire Disasters 2017;30(2):107–15.
5. Tripathee S, Basnet S. Epidemiology and outcome of hospitalized burn patients in tertiary care center in Nepal: two year retrospective study. Burns 2017;1(1):16–9.
6. Mann-Salinas EA, Baun MM, Meininger JC, et al. Novel predictors of sepsis outperform the American Burn Association sepsis criteria in the burn intensive care unit patient. J Burn Care Res 2013;34:31.
7. Schultz L, Walker SA, Elligsen M, et al. Identification of predictors of early infection in acute burn patients. Burns 2013;39:1355.
8. Jeschke MG, Gauglitz GG, Kulp GA, et al. Long-term persistence of the pathophysiologic response to severe burn injury. PLoS One 2011;6:e21245.
9. Greenhalgh D. Sepsis in the burn patient: a different problem than sepsis in the general population. Burns Trauma 2017;5:23. Available at: https://burnstrauma.biomedcentral.com/articles/10.1186/s41038-017-0089-5.
10. Fonseca J. Burn wound infections clinical presentation. 2016. Available at: https://emedicine.medscape.com/article/213595-clinical?pa=tXter9M8piyq26pHpmXMru EiP5ssNQiZvYObyq3fSHR%2FFc%2Fyz2VRpwJEq6zMRyjvJyGvMX%2Fu%2BWdl XoARf%2FT0zw%3D%3D.
11. van Duin D, Strassle PD, DiBiase LM, et al. Timeline of health care-associated infections and pathogens after burn injuries. Am J Infect Control 2016;44:1511.
12. Azzopardi EA, Azzopardi SM, Boyce DE, et al. Emerging gram-negative infections in burn wounds. J Burn Care Res 2011;32:570.
13. Yusuf K. Infection control in severely burned patients. World J Crit Care Med 2012;1(4):94–101.

Moving?

Make sure your subscription moves with you!

To notify us of your new address, find your **Clinics Account Number** (located on your mailing label above your name), and contact customer service at:

Email: journalscustomerservice-usa@elsevier.com

800-654-2452 (subscribers in the U.S. & Canada)
314-447-8871 (subscribers outside of the U.S. & Canada)

Fax number: 314-447-8029

Elsevier Health Sciences Division
Subscription Customer Service
3251 Riverport Lane
Maryland Heights, MO 63043

*To ensure uninterrupted delivery of your subscription,
please notify us at least 4 weeks in advance of move.